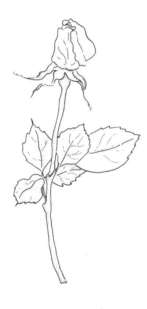

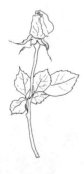

Essence of Love

By the same author:
Aromatherapy for Women

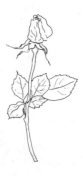

Essence of Love

Fragrance, Aphrodisiacs, and Aromatherapy for Lovers

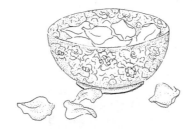

Maggie Tisserand

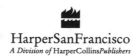

HarperSanFrancisco
A Division of HarperCollins*Publishers*

ESSENCE OF LOVE: *Fragrance, Aphrodisiacs, and Aromatherapy for Lovers.*
Copyright (c) 1993 by Maggie Tisserand. All rights reserved. Printed
in the United States of America. No part of this book may be used
or reproduced in any manner whatsoever without written permis-
sion except in the case of brief quotations embodied in critical arti-
cles and reviews. For information address HarperCollins Publishers,
10 East 53rd Street, New York, NY 10022.

Illustrations by Hilair Chism
Design by Margery Cantor

FIRST HARPERCOLLINS PAPERBACK EDITION PUBLISHED IN 1993

Library of Congress Cataloging–in–Publication Data
Tisserand, Maggie.
    Essence of love : fragrance, aphrodisiacs, and aromatherapy for
    lovers / Maggie Tisserand. – 1st HarperCollins pbk. ed.
        p. cm.
    Originally published: Thorsons, 1993.
    Includes bibliographical references and index.
    ISBN 0–06–250914–4
    1. Aromatherapy. 2. Aphrodisiacs. 3. Sex. I. Title.
RM666.A68T574 1994   93–31435
615'.321–dc20   CIP

            97 98 ❖ HAD 10 9 8 7 6 5 4 3 2

This book is dedicated to the lover within

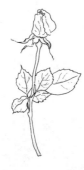

Contents

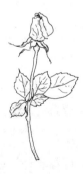

Acknowledgments

My grateful thanks go to the following people: Sue Robinson, for her support and assistance. Jane Graham–Maw, my editor, for her patience. Marek Urbanowitz, for his advice on Oriental medicine.

Thanks, too, to the researchers into the wonders of olfaction, whose findings have been quoted in chapter 7: Robert Ornstein and David Sobel, D. Michael Stoddart, Dietrich Gumbel, Max Lake, J. Mensing and C. Beck, Sigmund Freud, and Robert Holden.

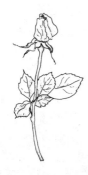

Introduction

The love of two pure lovers consists of desire
and in mutual pleasing. In it nothing can be
worthwhile unless their will be equal.

Jaufré Rudel

Sex is beautiful, fulfilling–and good exercise. No revelations
here; the benefits of good sex have been known and written
about for a long time. But what of the theory that sex can
improve your health, strengthen your immune system, and
prevent the onset of disease? When sex is enhanced by aromatherapy, all this is also true.

This is not a book on "how to get a man" or "how to score
with women." It is a book for lovers. You can be as hedonis-
tic as the ancient Greeks and Romans, as worshipful as the
Taoist Chinese or Tantric Hindu. The recipes and descriptions
in this book will help you use aromatic oils to scent and
massage your body and that of your partner. You can
indulge all your senses, in the privacy of the bedroom.

While writing this book I had to stop and ask myself "Why
am I writing a book about sex in this age of AIDS? Am I

exploring an issue thirty years out of date? Am I being irre-
sponsible?" A bit of reflection, however, gave me my answer.
There is no reason for sex to stop being fun just because it
needs to be 'safe.' And isn't the safest sex that which takes
place within a loving monogamous relationship? Monogamy
need never be boring. Sex need never be boring: each of us
has an innate need for pleasure and fulfillment, as well as a
need to give pleasure to another. What greater or keener
pleasure is there than that of sex?

Sex and aromatherapy marry together perfectly. Imagine
how, hundreds and even thousands of years ago, lovers
rubbed scented oils onto each other's body, experiencing the
fulfillment of all their senses. Their sense of smell delighted in
the wonderful perfume of natural essences intermingling with
the body's own perfume; their sense of touch revelled in the
feel of massaging their loved one or in being massaged by
him or her; their eyes beheld the erotic sight of oil glistening
on naked skin; their ears took in spoken words of pleasure–
and when they kissed, the fifth sense was fulfilled, for what
finer taste is there than that of the lips of your lover?

I believe that good sex is life–enhancing, as is aromatherapy. Even when sexual intercourse is not involved, the physical pleasure of touching, of intimate body contact in the form
of massage–all this equals happiness, and happiness is a

potent medicine. Joy and pleasure send the right stimuli to the body cells to keep them healthy. By using essential oils on a daily basis we create within ourselves a state of health and harmony.

You may already be a keen advocate of aromatherapy and appreciate its benefits, but if this book is your introduction to essential oils, you have a treat in store. Enjoy the sensual pleasures that lie ahead. Fragrant essences not only excite the senses and lift the emotions but also work on a deeper level, to nourish and protect the cells of the body.

Aromatherapy can be used to address many health problems, enabling us, for example, to break with the antibiotic habit. In recent years, researcher Clive Wood has looked at the connection between mind, brain, and the immune system. He calls this study *psycho-neuro-immunology*. We know, for instance, that people can truly die of a broken heart–such is the power of our emotions on our physical being. Surely we must also be able to use this power to maintain a strong and healthy body.

Aromatherapy can also bring about a peaceful state of mind, which in itself can bring harmony to a relationship. Many Eastern texts, when referring to meditation, stress the importance of deep breathing. They say that the mind follows the breath. Within our polluted environment we tend to be shallow breathers. When experiencing a delightful aromatherapy massage or when soaking in a deliciously fragrant bath, we automatically take deeper breaths to savour the beauty of the scents around us.

In this book I have tried to present practical tips and recipes and alternative methods of treating sexual problems as well as offering a brief history of the erotic use of aromatics since ancient times. I have also discussed the theory that inside every woman there exist attributes of several goddesses. Aphrodite, being the goddess of love and sensuality, is the one this book is most interested in revealing. By letting go of fears and preconditioning, and using essential oils with imagination and confidence, every woman can allow this part of herself to emerge and flourish.

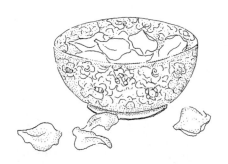

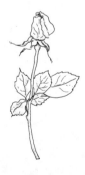

Chapter 1

Aromatherapy for Life

Sex puts a sparkle in the eye, a glow
to the cheeks and makes the world
seem like a better place.

Mantak Chia, *Taoist Secrets of Love*

Few of us would argue with this sentiment,
yet it's easy to let the pressures and problems
of modern living dampen our desire, making
us "not in the mood," preferring the television to
a night of lovemaking.

We have become too used to obtaining objects of desire—
cars, holidays, custom kitchens—merely by signing an "easy
credit" contract. This habit of instant gratification can influence the way we view our sexual needs. We may believe what
we see in films and read in the press, magazines, and books:
that sex—any kind of sex—is the answer. One-night stands, extramarital affairs, or simply choosing partners for their sexy
image are all seen as ways of fulfilling our fundamental need
for intimacy. But are they really?

Holistic Sex

Many of us recognize holistic medicine as a safe and effective system that takes an overview of the *whole* person–his or her lifestyle, diet, and mental outlook as well as medical and hereditary history and total symptom picture. In the same way, holistic sex brings together every aspect of sexual union: the physical, mental, and emotional. Sex therapist and author Barbara de Angelis writes, "the sexual act is so powerful because it is the closest we ever come to uniting with another human being. If that physical union is not balanced and matched by emotional closeness, the same act that can be so full of joy becomes one that leaves [us] feeling isolated, lonely and unfulfilled." Psychologist Erich Fromm puts it this way: "Sex [without love] becomes a desperate attempt to escape the anxiety engendered by separateness, and it results in an ever-increasing sense of separateness, since the sexual act without love never bridges the gap between two human beings, except momentarily."

Holistic sex is the mix of all three types of loving, so that we love and want our partners on a physical, mental, and emotional level. Or, to put it another way, we lust after their body, thinking about them turns us on, and we bond with them

2

emotionally. We love their mind, body, and spirit with our mind, body, and spirit:

> When their bodies merge into each other, desire can turn into joy, and physical lust and its gratification can become an expression of unconditional devotion which pervades mind, body and spirit.
>
> Erich Fromm, *The Art of Loving*

Physical, mental, and emotional—this is the ideal sexual mix, and within the mix are all the ingredients for a lasting and happy relationship. Holistic sex is as valid to our emotional health and happiness as holistic medicine is to our physical and mental health. And aromatherapy has its part to play in this mix. Beautiful aromas act on all three aspects of our being, and can be used in obvious and more subtle ways.

Inner Sex

In the 1970s Timothy Gallway wrote a fascinating book called *The Inner Game of Tennis*. His hypothesis was that to be centered and "in the now" puts us in contact with a higher power that

3

knows instinctively what to do. Although written for tennis players, the basic message can be adopted by lovers–something inside you knows how to love, and the love is always there, irrespective of whether you currently have a partner. When you fall in love with someone, the feelings of love do not come from the other person but from within you.

Erich Fromm writes, "Respect for one's own integrity and uniqueness, love for and understanding of one's own self, cannot be separated from respect and love and understanding for another individual." He understood that we need first to love ourselves before we can truly love another, because in order to give we must feel we are rich enough in love to be generous with our love. If you are tired or depressed you cannot give. You need to take care of yourself first, utilizing the essential oils that will cleanse, uplift, heal, and energize your body and emotions. Only when your cup is full can it overflow to others.

> The inner smile is the recipe for living in simple harmony with yourself and others. The inner smile is the smile of total happiness. This is not the social smile. This smile rises from the cells and organs of the body.
>
> Mantak Chia, *Taoist Secrets of Love*

4

What Is Aromatherapy?

Aromatherapy uses the essential oils of plants to heal and beautify the body. Connected to herbal medicine but having its own separate identity, aromatherapy takes aromatic plant material such as basil or lavender and distills its essence, then uses this essence in numerous beneficial ways.

Imagine how, thousands of years ago, humans watched wild horses running free across the plains and marveled at their beauty and awe-inspiring speed. If someone were lucky enough to catch one by surprise, he or she would experience the speed, power, and majesty of riding, but as soon as one dismounted the horse would be gone. Then one day humans invented rope and made a lasso. They began to catch these wild, free animals, taming them and harnessing their power.

Now imagine how, thousands of years ago, humans beheld the glory of the aromatic plant kingdom, rejoicing in the scent of the rose, for example. Yet people could not capture its exquisite fragrance. Then, one day, distillation was invented and the fragrance of the rose was captured forevermore, to be enjoyed at any time of the day or night–any month of the year.

Distillation is the rope that lassos the aromas of flowers and plants, so that their power is harnessed for our purposes.

However, aromatherapy is far more than just the experience of a pleasant aroma; it is not by chance that "therapy" is part of the word. For here, in using essential oils from plants, we have at our disposal many choices: we have fragrances that can lift our emotions–transporting us from depression to happiness; healing essences that work with our bodies to combat illness and disease; and aromas that can provide us with untold sensual pleasures.

Essences and the Emotions

How we cope in times of stress can greatly influence our general health. Our ability to "weather the storm" makes all the difference between drowning in a sea of overwhelming emotion or calmly sailing through the troughs and peaks of life. In times of trouble aromatherapy can help. Just a few drops of clary sage oil on a room fragrancer or added to the bath will soon restore mental clarity.

Illness often causes depression as it interrupts the flow of what we normally expect to do–which is to be active and useful. Healing and recovery can be hindered by a depressed state, as mental depression also causes a depression of the immune system. Use any of the uplifting essences–rose, ylang ylang, lavender, bergamot, geranium, rosewood, rosemary, sandalwood, neroli, or petigrain–to remove unnecessary burdens from the body and allow it to repair itself.

Our "will" is a powerful tool that we can use for our own benefit and for the benefit of others, but only if we recognize that we own such a tool. Willpower is linked to the solar plexus, and when we are under attack from negative emotions, whether our own or someone else's, the solar plexus area becomes very tender. It is a vulnerable and highly sensitive area of the body, and is where "gut feelings" are registered. Overloading this area can result in loss of willpower, a feeling of helplessness, and the inability to effect positive change.

"I feel as though I have been punched in the gut" is a familiar cry from someone who has suffered an emotional shock, as is the expression "I'm gutted." Diluted essential oils, when applied to the solar plexus, can help to heal and protect this susceptible region.

Beauty Inside and Out

Because of their beneficial action on the skin, essential oils make perfect skin care products. Valuable research into this area has been conducted by Dietrich Gumbel. He says that "blood sugars, which have been stored in fat deposits, are released by the use of sandalwood [oil], so that the sugars can reach the skin and oxidize, thus vitalizing the skin. Skin water–retention is improved and the elasticity of fibers is maintained." In other words, sandalwood helps your skin stay moisturized and young–looking, from within.

Lavender, rose, bergamot, rosewood, and ylang ylang are in-valuable if you want to maintain a healthy, glowing complex-ion. Acne and even chronic skin problems such as eczema and psoriasis can be treated successfully with soothing essential oils.

Tea tree, lemon, lavender, and geranium regulate the skin's production of sebaceous oils, and so can help treat greasy hair. And a combination of tea tree oil and the "liquid wax" of the jojoba plant makes for a very effective treatment for dandruff. More on aromatherapy for healthy and beautiful skin and hair can be found in chapter 5.

Staying in Tune

Aromatherapy self–help can strengthen our bodies and pro-tect us from succumbing to colds, flu, and other diseases. Oils that help to fight viral and bacterial infections include laven-der, ravansara, niaouli, bergamot, tea tree, lemon, and myrtle. Any one of these, diluted in a base oil, may be massaged into your back and chest to help you to feel better. With the possi-ble exception of tea tree (which cannot be said to be pleasant-smelling), any of the other oils makes a wonderfully soothing and healthy bath. As only 4–6 drops are required for a therapeutic bath, using essential oils is also a very economic way of staying healthy.

Blends of these essences can be made following the instructions in chapter 8. More detailed information on the use of essential oils for curing common ailments can be found in my book *Aromatherapy for Women*.

The Goddess Within

Over the centuries gender roles have shifted; what is expected of women has changed dramatically; more importantly, the way women view themselves and their position in society and in relationships has altered drastically. Today's woman is multifaceted, often juggling a career, husband, children, politics, the pursuit of sports, and much else besides.

In a remarkable book called *The Goddess Within*, psychologists Jennifer and Roger Woolger attribute these different facets of a woman's psyche to six major goddesses: Demeter, the nurturer; Hera, the power-seeker; Athena, the wise and confident career woman; Artemis, the lover of Nature and freedom; Persephone, the intuitive, psychic, sensitive aspect of a woman; and of course Aphrodite, goddess of love, ruler over sensuality, the arts, and beauty in all things.

9

The balance between these different goddesses will vary from woman to woman and even from time to time within one woman when her lifestyle forces her to embrace one goddess more fully. As the authors of this marvelous book say, "To know oneself more fully as a woman is to know which goddess one is primarily ruled by and to be aware of how different goddesses influence the various stages and turning points of one's life."

For aromatherapy, it is Aphrodite particularly who interests us. She is the goddess governing perfumery, sensuality, massage, cosmetics, and all things aesthetic and joyful. Being ashamed of your sexuality means that you are not sufficiently in touch with the Aphrodite part of yourself.

Aromatherapy can help you to get and stay in touch with this element of your psyche; oils such as rose or myrtle can help you to identify with this goddess within. You share with all women an innate sensuality, and should rejoice in it. You may be a partner, mother, co-worker, but you are also a vibrant, sexy, sensual being.

In Greek myth, myrtle was the plant chosen by Aphrodite to hide her nakedness and it has been associated with her ever since. To let go of your business stresses, domestic strains, mental worries, or physical aches and pains and connect with the loving, sensual woman within, take a myrtle bath in a quiet, subtly lit room. Imagine that you are free from your current problems, and allow yourself to be enveloped in this timeless fragrance as it cleanses, soothes, and inspires you. Allow your imagination to make you feel that you are a goddess—after all, you are breathing the same aromas as the goddess did, all those millennia ago.

Rose oil is soothing to the heart and comforting in times of sorrow; through its uplifting powers, it removes psychological pain and opens up a channel to sensitivity, love, and empathy. It balances a woman's hormonal system and would be useful for anyone who feels "at a distance" from her emotional center.

Using geranium and clary sage oils will help to harmonize a body that has been neglected and is tense and lacking in sensitivity, whether male or female. When you become aggressive and full of stress, a massage using clary sage, rose, myrtle, or geranium will rebalance the male/female forces within you, resulting in a calmer, more lovable you.

When the pressures of holding down a job or the trauma of losing a job have temporarily "castrated" you, and the joy of making love seems like a distant memory, then once again aromatherapy can be of assistance. Using those aromatics that

11

contain phytohormones (plant hormones) can restore harmony to your body and mind, leading to a calmer way of being, and allowing you to accept help and healing from those around you. Being in harmony and being in touch with yourself brings about the ability to empathize with and reach out to others in their time of suffering.

The Greek god Apollo, representing life, immortality, harmonious balance, beauty, and goodness, could be considered to be the male version of Aphrodite. The way to become the perfect lover is to be beautiful from the inside out–and allowing aromatic essences to make you feel beautiful is a step in the right direction.

> *Of all the ten thousand things created by heaven,*
> *man is the most precious.*
> *Of all the things that make man prosper, none can*
> *be compared to sexual intercourse.*

Li Tung Hsuan,
Ars Amatoria (The Art of the
Bedchamber)

Chapter 2

An Erotic History

> Therefore I come forth to meet thee, diligent-
> ly to seek thy face, and I have found thee. I
> have decked my bed with coverings of
> tapestry, with carved works, with fine linen
> of Egypt. I have perfumed my bed with
> myrrh, aloes, and cinnamon. Come, let us
> take our fill of love until morning, let us
> solace ourselves with love.
>
> Proverbs 7

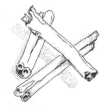

The word *aromatherapy* may have been coined in the twenti-
eth century, but the use of aromatic oils and unguents for
religious and sexual purposes goes back thousands of years,
to the dawn of civilization.

It is difficult to pinpoint which civilization first had the
knowledge of perfumery and aromatherapy. The ancient
Chinese say that The Yellow Emperor first brought medicine
and perfumes to the world, while in India the birth of perfumery is attributed to the god Indra. Most probably the art

of aromatherapy passed on like this: ancient China/India →
Egyptians/Hebrews → Greeks → Romans → throughout the
Roman Empire/Arab world → on to Europe/rest of the world.

Wherever aromatics were grown, people recognized their
contribution to sexual and religious ecstasy and, realizing the
value of these commodities, traveled to other lands to trade,
selling the aromatic plants that grew in their own land and
buying aromatics that did not. In this way the knowledge of
perfumery/aromatherapy spread.

Aromatherapy Through the Ages

Scent and Sex in Ancient China and Japan

Sexual union between man and woman was the basic concept
behind Yin and Yang, the ancient Chinese polar and comple-
mentary forces of life. The Chinese believed that sexual union
had a cosmic influence on world events. Earthquakes, tidal
waves, fierce winds–all these were attributable to disharmony.
The emperor and empress of China epitomized the balance of
the positive and negative elements in the realm. Special court
ladies kept records (with a special red writing brush) of the
sexual relations between the emperor and his wives. According
to R. H. Gulik, "ancient China considered the clouds to be
earth's ova, which are fertilized by the rain, heaven's sperm."

The emperor had one wife, with whom he copulated once a month. He would practice the Taoist discipline of having sex without ejaculating, which allowed him to indulge in sexual relations many times in the space of one night. Although he only had sex with his wife once a month, he also had three consorts, nine wives of second rank, twenty-seven wives of third rank, and eighty-one concubines. Conserving his sperm was the only way in which he could make love with these 121 different women! Far from being exhausted by so much activity, the Chinese recognized that "during sexual union the man's vital force is fed and strengthened by that of the woman, supposed to reside in her vaginal secretions."

Old Chinese sexual guidebooks preach that the more times one has sex without ejaculating the greater the benefits to the health. Once—and the vital essences are strengthened; twice—there will be an improvement in sight and hearing; three times—and all diseases will be cured; further practice will result in the man's having a religious experience. By recycling the semen it was thought that the brain would be nourished and that longevity would be assured.

In their time these sex manuals would have played another very important role—that of mentally exciting the emperor, for it would not be possible for him to feel aroused by each of his women when he needed to make love with at least

15

three every day of the week. Yin and Yang depended upon the harmony between a man and a woman, and as a woman is slower to be aroused and to reach orgasm than a man, it would be up to him to preserve the harmony and satisfy her needs by practicing "The Tao of Loving": "Man is fire, which quickly flares up and can easily be extinguished. Woman is water, which takes longer to heat up, but once hot, cools down slowly. Fire is extinguished by water and water is heated by fire."

At the same time it was recognized that inside every man there was some feminine and inside every woman there was some masculine. Harmony between the two is only possible if the man is in harmony with himself and the woman in harmony with herself. Having found harmony within himself, the man could practice Taoist sex, making love to his chosen partner for several hours at a time, without expending his ejaculate.

Many Chinese herbs, such as ginseng, were useful in strengthening sexual potency; aromatic spices and herbs were used regularly both to enhance sexual union and to promote harmony between the two partners.

Such was the Japanese understanding of the importance of sexual expression that the genitals were worshiped. Ancient fertility festivals frequently culminated in a sexual free-for-all. Phallic worship is one of the oldest aspects of religion in

Japan, and even today a shrine exists in Kanamara with a giant wooden phallus on which grandmothers sit their small granddaughters in the hope that they will receive good luck for a fertile and happy marriage.

Courtship rituals were often elaborate affairs, with go-betweens carrying letters and poems. Sometimes a poem would be written on tinted paper, according to the season of the year, and delivered on a heavily scented fan. If the correspondence was mutually encouraging, it would result in the suitor making a night call to the woman. "Stealing behind the curtains and into the scented darkness of the waiting lady's bedchamber, the man simply removed his clothing and got into bed with her" (Nicholas Bornoff, *Pink Samurai*). Sex was guiltlessly regarded as one of the pleasures of life–and free love was very common-place. Attached to the kimono sashes of both sexes were little boxes called *Inro*. These were used for medicines and love potions and other aids to sexual fulfillment.

The Japanese passion for incense was transformed into an art still practiced today by devotees of Kodo and known as the Way of Incense. In ancient times perfumes would waft through the temples, clothing, and people's homes, and of course bathwater was delicately scented. Bathing in Japan was and still is a very important ritual. Washing was done first outside the bath, and only after scrubbing away the dirt

17

and dead skin debris and rinsing thoroughly did the bather step into the deliciously scented tub of water, where the cares of the day were gently soothed away.

Tantric Sex

Tantra, or Tantric, sex is the Indian equivalent of Taoist sex. The major difference is that Tantra is seen to be a step on the road to spiritual enlightenment and mystical union, whereas practicing Taoist sex does not require a belief system, merely the cultivation of willpower.

The Hindu words for the genital organs are *lingam* for the man and *yoni* for the woman, and these organs—which to us are associated with sex, birth, and maturity—have in Indian culture a much more spiritual association. Just as the Christian theory of the origin of the world is the Garden of Eden, Adam and Eve, so in India the god Shiva and his mighty lingam are believed to have brought the world into existence. Throughout India there are shrines—elaborate ones in temples and simpler ones tucked away on side streets—where the lingam and yoni can be worshiped. Sex in all its forms is considered acceptable and beautiful.

A nation that reveres the sex organs certainly has no sexual hang-ups compared to Western nations, and India's openness to and unabashed enjoyment of sex has provided the world with the most famous sex manual of all–the *Kama Sutra*. This text's illustrations of the various sex postures are not considered pornographic, nor is its discussion of oral sex meant to be taboo but a normal part of healthy lovemaking. Yet eye contact is still considered the most important facet of lovemaking, because the eyes are windows to the soul, and *Tantra* is the experience of God within oneself and within one's partner, through sexual union.

Perfumes, particularly sandalwood, went easily from the temple to the bedchamber. The Hindu god Indra is always represented with his breast tinged with sandalwood. Kama, Hindu god of love, is always pictured holding a bow and arrow. The bow is made of sugar cane, the string consists of bees, and each of his five arrows is tipped with the blossom of a flower. The arrows are meant to pierce the heart of the recipient through one of his or her five senses. One arrow is tipped with the jasmine flower, known for its aphrodisiacal value. *Kama Sutra*, or Kama Shastri, means "Scripture of Love," as *Kama* is the Hindu word for love and is the equivalent of Eros or Cupid. The *Kama Sutra* has many references to aromatics, as they were an intrinsic part of the sexual act:

> ... the outer room, balmy with rich perfumes,
> should contain a bed, soft, agreeable to the sight,
> covered with a clean white cloth, low in the middle

part, having garlands and bunches of flowers upon
it, and a canopy above it, and two pillows, one at
the top, another at the bottom. There should also
be a sort of couch besides and at the head of this a
sort of stool, on which should be placed the fragrant ointments for the night, as well as flowers . . .
and other fragrant substances.

The *Ananga Ranga*, another Indian text, rivals the *Kama Sutra*
and gives the following recipe for a night of passion:

. . . scattered about this apartment, place musical
instruments, bottles of rose-water and various
essences . . . Both man and woman should contend
against any reserve, or false shame, giving themselves up in complete nakedness to unrestrained
voluptuousness, upon a high and handsome bed-
stead; the sheets being sprinkled with flowers,
such as aloes and other fragrant woods. In such a
place, let the man, ascending the throne of love,
enjoy the woman in ease and comfort, gratifying
his and her every wish and every whim.

A lovely story illustrating the use of perfumes to seduce a
woman comes from *The Perfumed Garden*, written by Sheik
Nefzawi late in the fourteenth century:

Two prophets lived at the same time, and Sheja, the prophetess, wrote a letter to Mosailama, refuting his right to call himself a prophet. Mosailama sought advice from his counselors, who recommended that he invite Sheja for a meeting to discuss their problem. In preparation for Sheja's arrival, Mosailama was to erect a tent of colored brocade on the outskirts of town, and then "fill it with delicious perfumes of various kinds, amber, musk and scented flowers such as the rose, orange blossom, jonquil, jasmine, hyacinth, pink, and others similar. That done you will place in the tent golden cassolettes filled with perfumes . . . Then the tent must be closed so that none of the perfume can escape, and when the vapors have become sufficiently intense to impregnate the water which is in the tent, you will mount your throne and send for the prophetess, who will remain with you in the tent alone. When she inhales the perfumes she will be delighted, all her joints will slacken and she will swoon away. After having possessed her you will be spared trouble from her." When everything was in order Mosailama sent for Sheja, who quickly became stupefied and began to lose her presence of mind.

Instead of discussing their conflicts, Mosailama knew he could have his way with her and asked "Whatever posture you prefer, speak, and you will be satisfied." "I want it all ways," replied the prophetess, thus bringing to a satisfactory end the dispute between the two prophets.

As much credence was given to the rejuvenating properties of aromatic plants as to their seductive powers.

"If you wish to repeat the act, perfume yourself with sweet odors, then approach the woman and you will attain a happy result" (*Kama Sutra*).

"He who will feed for several days on eggs cooked with myrrh, cinnamon, and pepper will find an increased vigor in his erections and in his capacity for coition" (*The Perfumed Garden*). Little wonder that these "scriptures of love" were written in a part of the world where sun and sex were a daily delight, where sandalwood trees grew in abundance, otto of roses was distilled, and hundreds of aromatic spices, grasses, and flowers were a part of everyday life.

Ancient Egyptians and Hebrews

It is from India, as well as from China, that the ancient Egyptians obtained their knowledge and their supplies of many aromatics. The Egyptians were the inventors of the public baths, later borrowed by the Romans and adopted as their own.

After their daily ablutions the Egyptians would rub themselves all over with fragrant oils and ointments. The unguents used were many and varied and were primarily dispensed by the priests, who alone were acquainted with the mysteries of the compounding art. From the priests, who could be called the first perfumers, the skills were learned by the temple attendants and then by ordinary members of the populace. It must be remembered that a perfume and a medicine were one and the same to the ancient Egyptians. In the time of the Pharaohs, Egyptian women appreciated the value of perfumes for sexual attraction and hundreds of formulations were known. Perfumes were used to camouflage body odors, to scent the homes and public meeting places, and to fragrance the hair and even the genitalia.

The passion for perfumes continued to increase in Egypt until the time of Cleopatra, when it can be said to have reached its apex. Queen Cleopatra used aromatics in a lavish way, which may have been a contributing factor to her active sex life. As well as being lover to Julius Caesar and Mark Anthony, she is said to have fellated 100 centurions in a single day! Certainly she was no novice in the art of seduction: when summoned by Mark Anthony to meet him on the banks of the Tiber, she drenched the sails of her barge with jasmine and other heavy sensual aromatics. Having sailed to where he waited, she invited Mark Anthony on board. "The very winds were lovesick," Shakespeare writes in *Anthony and Cleopatra*, and this may account for the fact that Mark Anthony was completely spellbound by Cleopatra, to the exclusion of all duties and obligations to his country.

Hebrews were kept as slaves in Egypt, and after their release brought the arts of perfumery to their own people. Perfume was one of the means of seduction resorted to by Judith when she sought Holofernes in his tent, determined to liberate her people from his oppression. Elsewhere in the Old Testament the Queen of Sheba and King Solomon act out their erotic and aromatic fantasy: "My lover has the scent of myrrh, he shall lie all night on my breasts." Other known aphrodisiacs are mentioned in Proverbs: "I have perfumed my bed with myrrh, aloes, and cinnamon."

Greek Gods and Roman Emperors

Many beautiful and romantic stories describe the origin of aromatic use, and none is more beguiling than the Greek version.

The goddess Aphrodite arose from the waves and, realizing her nakedness, plucked some sprigs from a myrtle bush to cover herself. This is why, it is said, the myrtle plant has leaves shaped like a vagina, the outer lips (labia majora) being likened to "the lips of the myrtle" and the inner (labia minora) to "the fruit of the myrtle." Aphrodite was worshiped as the goddess of love, beauty, sexuality, and passion; she ruled all things sensual, including the knowledge of the sexual use of aromatic plants. From her name we have the word aphrodisiac; her son's name, Eros, gives us "erotic."

According to Greek legend the art of perfumery came to mortals when Aphrodite's handmaiden, Oenone, confided in her lover, Paris. Paris, after anointing himself with aromatics, managed to steal Helen of Troy away from her husband, Menelaus. When Helen eventually returned to Greece she brought with her the knowledge of perfumery. Another of Helen's lovers, Alexandros, was saved from the clutches of the jealous Menelaus by Aphrodite, who "snatched him away with the ease of a god, wrapped him in thick mist, and set him down in his sweetly-scented bedroom." Aphrodite then united the lovers: "She took hold of Helen's sweet-smelling dress and twitched it with her hand. 'Come this way, Alexandros is calling you back to the house. He is there in the bedroom, on the carved bed, shining in his own beauty.' "

Aphrodite was not always so kind, for when the women of Lemnos refused to pay homage to her she cursed them with a foul smell which made their husbands turn away from them.

In despair and frustration they massacred their menfolk and lived empty, celibate lives until Jason and the Argonauts arrived on the island during a tempestuous storm. So desperate for sex were these women of Lemnos that they bartered hospitality for lovemaking, but to enable this to take place they first had to burn vast quantities of incense on the altar of Aphrodite, not only to appease the goddess but so the sensual odors would mask the foul smell they'd been cursed with.

Ancient Greeks colonized parts of Italy; in Sybaris the men and women bathed several times a day in aromatic water and it was this indulgence in the physical pleasures that gave us the word *sybaritic*. Later when the Romans began to amass their Empire, conquering Southern Italy, the knowledge of perfumery passed to Rome.

The Roman goddess of love and sensuality was Venus, and she too was supposed to have been born from the sea and to have covered her nakedness with myrtle leaves. The Three Graces in attendance on Venus and her son, Cupid, were crowned with myrtle leaves; when accompanying The Muses, however, they wore wreaths of roses. Rose essence was called "the blood of Venus" and Roman temples were always adorned with roses. Venus gave us the word *venery*, meaning sexual desire, and *venereal* (of the sexual organs), and it is not coincidence that Venice is called "city of lovers."

Roman feasts in honor of Bacchus, god of wine and lust, were elaborate occasions, with roses being as important a commodity as wine, women, and food. The Romans were obsessed by the rose. Rose water perfumed the public baths, flowed from fountains in the emperor's palaces, and were strewn everywhere at banquets. Even wine was rose–scented– and the cure for overindulgence? Rose water.

Although not the earliest aromatherapists, the Romans knew that perfumes in general possessed medicinal properties. The most popular recipes were inscribed on marble tablets in the temple of Venus. Brides-to-be in the fourth century B.C. were anointed with aromatic oils prior to their wedding. Romans borrowed from the Egyptians the use of the public bath, which they would visit daily. Ovid, the great poet in the time of the Emperor Augustus, told the Romans, "Adonis is a woodland boy, but became the darling of Venus. It is by simple cleanliness that you should seek to attract . . ." Rome in Nero's time had over 1,000 *unctuaria* (baths that specialized in the use of fragrances). Nero's wife, Poppaea, bathed in scented ass's milk. She was a poet, and wrote, "Wives are out of fashion now/Mistresses are in/Rose leaves are dated/Now cinnamon's the thing." Eating, drinking, bathing, and copulating were not only indulged in but actually worshiped. One month in every year male genitals were

worshiped in honor of the god Liber. The month of this phallic worship corresponded to the time of year ruled by Libra.
Romans worshiped the genitals as the gateway to immortality
both for their procreative powers and because it was believed
that one could attain spiritual union with the gods by reach-
ing sexual heights of ecstasy, as was believed by those who
practiced the Indian *Tantra*.

Byzantium

Wherever we look in history and see how the mighty empires
rose and fell, we can see evidence of aromatics used for sensual pleasures. After the fall of the Roman Empire, power
passed to the Eastern Empire, as Byzantium became the hub
of trade. Harem women relied heavily on the use of aromatics–for their beauty, their ability to satisfy their master sexually, and to appease their boredom during the long, hot days
with nothing better to do than prepare for a night of lovemaking. Spices such as cloves and ginger were rubbed onto
the body, because the women of the harem believed that
these aromatics had the ability to increase sexual power.

Bathing was not only a necessary obligation but the main
social event of the day, where dozens of nude beauties whiled
away the hours. The bathing ritual lasted for several hours,
and afterwards "they at once spring upon their sofas, where

the attentive slaves fold them in warm clothes, and pour essences upon their hair, which they twist loosely without attempting to dislodge the wet ... and then cover with handsome handkerchiefs or embroidered muslin ... perfumed water is scattered over the face and hands, and the exhausted bather sinks into a luxurious slumber beneath a coverlet of satin or eider down."

Europe and the New World

In Europe perfume, although introduced by the Romans, went out of fashion and was only really reintroduced when the Crusaders returned from their travels and their wives found themselves competing with the seductive memories their husbands brought home with them. Exotic perfumes brought home by the Crusaders became popular with the women, who took to wearing perfume in an attempt to lay the ghosts of Arabian nights to rest and so to regain their husbands' affections.

"With the Renaissance the perfumer's art was revived with a vengeance ... it was also acceptable once more for men and women to search openly for the erotic." Catherine de Medici adored aromatics, especially neroli, which she transplanted

29

from her native Italy to the South of France when she became wife of Henry II. Despite the fact that Diane de Poitiers was the young and beautiful mistress of the king, Catherine managed to give him five heirs.

The Empress Josephine loved scents, and being a Creole brought up in Martinique she was used to wearing oils and creams of almond and coconut imbued with heady aromas from jasmine and other heavily scented flowers. She was fanatical about the use of aromatics and impregnated the walls of her bedroom with musk. Her favorite flower was the violet. Napoleon gave her instructions to wear only orange water, lavender water, and eau de Cologne when she visited him on location, claiming that her perfumes distracted him to such an extent that he could not concentrate on planning his battle strategies. But when they had been apart for a lengthy period he would send word to her: "Je reviens en trois jours, ne te laves pas" (I return in three days, don't wash), so potent did he find her natural body odors. When Josephine died Napoleon had violets planted on her tomb, and in loving memory of their nights of passion he wore a pressed violet in the gold locket which he wore constantly round his neck.

Though pomanders were originally used for medicinal purposes, in the seventeenth century many upper-class European women wore them solely as a means of enveloping themselves in an aura of perfume, in order to attract the attentions of a lover. Perfumed bracelets became popular as, it was believed, they "by their odiferous scent conduce much, to the making your captives numerous, though they bind only your arms, yet they take men your prisoners."

The use of aromatics for seduction became so rife in Europe that the English Parliament of 1770 even passed an act intended to protect men from being beguiled into marriage by the fairer sex. "All women, of whatever age . . . that shall from and after such act, impose upon, seduce and betray in matrimony, any of his subjects, by the use of scents, paints, cosmetics. . . . shall incur the penalty of the law in force against witchcraft and like misdemeanors and that marriage shall stand null and void." Witch-hunts and the Puritanism of Cromwell's reign did much to destroy the love of perfumes, sensual pleasures, and open sexuality. During the Restoration perfumes made a comeback and one popular scent was an orange fragrance created in memory of Nell Gwynne, mistress of Charles II, as her humble origins were that of an orange-seller.

Elsewhere around the globe people were also employing aromatics in their love lives. Women in Senegal used the tubers of the ginger plant to make belts, with the aim of arousing the dormant senses of their men. In North America, Native American tribes made a tea from juniper berries, which they drank as a contraceptive. At wedding rituals great bowls of yucca suds (aloe vera) were prepared so that the bride and groom could ceremonially wash each other's head.

Every civilization has employed aromatics in the course of a fulfilling sex life, and only in times of repression and fear has the use and appreciation of sensual aromatics been lost.

> Man only doth smell and take delight in the odors of flowers and sweet things. Sweet scents are the sweet vehicles of still sweeter thoughts.
>
> Walter Landor

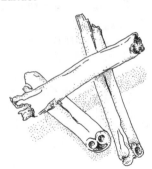

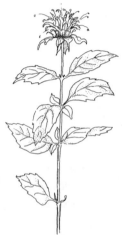

Chapter 3

Lasting Impressions

He found her as she slept in the beauty of her palace. She awakened at the fragrance of the god, which she smelled in the presence of his majesty. When he came before her, she rejoiced in the sight of his beauty. His love passed into her limbs, which the fragrance of the god flooded.

From an inscription on the
chamber wall of an Egyptian pyramid

Enhancing Your Natural Body Scent

Each of us has our own "smell," which is as unique as our fingerprints. Mostly we are unable to detect it ourselves because our noses become satiated with one smell after a short period of time–just as when we apply perfume and cannot smell it after half an hour even though other people can be aware of it for many hours. Uniquely personal, we can often only detect our own scent when we take a worn item of clothing from the back of the wardrobe and realize that it needs laundering. This is our "stale" scent, however, an aroma we find disagreeable and do not choose to be associated with; yet our "fresh" scent signature is one that we take with us wherever we go and by which we are recognizably ourselves.

Smell has very strong erotic connotations, and we can be attracted to or repelled by another person by the way he or she smells. Just as you can love someone for the softness of their skin, so you can love someone for the smell of it. Part of loving someone is loving their smell, and "just as it may be difficult to live with someone whose voice is unpleasantly loud or shrill, so it may be impossible to live with someone whose body smell is disagreeable." Some North African tribes give so much credence to personal aroma that the wife can be instantly divorced if she does not smell "right."

Your individual aroma can be affected by what you put into your system—food, alcohol, coffee and other strong drink, cigar or cigarette smoke, and so forth—and by your mental and spiritual attitudes. Anger or fear, for example, can alter your smell as your body releases adrenaline. In an acute situation this chemical change may be insignificant, but if it becomes chronic due to the pressures of work, then your body chemistry can be altered to such a degree that your partner no longer "recognizes" the person with whom he or she fell in love.

Acupuncturists are trained to recognize different body smells, and so are able to utilize the sense of smell as a diagnostic tool. Spiritual harmony is supposed to imbue the body with a beautiful aroma, and reports from India claim that after the death of holy men there is sometimes a lingering aroma of beautiful blossoms.

It is interesting to note that the Japanese, who have long employed a daily relaxing bath in scented water, do not have an underarm smell–there are of course a few exceptions, but in general their understanding of the need to create harmony in their everyday lives, and their conscious effort "not to disturb the *wa*" (harmony) may have caused a systematic physiological change over the passage of time.

Sexual excitement causes all sorts of exotic odors to emanate from the body–from the breath, the skin, and in particular the genitalia. In many successful relationships the partners are able to recognize each other's smells, as the body's natural perfume is indeed a potent method of nonverbal communication. An experiment showing that when a woman's vaginal secretions were applied to her chest she and her partner had sex more often has recently been reported in the *British Journal of Sexual Medicine*; further research into a woman's intimate smells has revealed that men prefer the aroma of the vagina at the time of ovulation.

Sexual excitement causes the skin, breath, nipples, and sexual organs to release exotic odors, and these "natural body perfumes" can be enhanced by the subtle use of essential oils. Courtesans of medieval Europe used to wear a little of their vaginal secretion as perfume, dabbing it behind their ears and on their necks–and found it to be a powerful sex attractant.

Understanding of the link between sensuality and fragrance has long been exploited by the world's perfume houses, although marketing is subject to current fashion. Maurice Roger, Dior's top perfumer, says, "The idea of sensual femininity is a phenomenon of our contemporary society, and the way one expresses sensuality depends on the evolution of culture. What is happening now is a softer mood where a woman's personality can shine through her fragrance instead of her having to rent something from outside. Sensuality now is not a vulgar emission of sex-symbol sexuality, but a blend of character and spirit."

The sense of smell has been linked to the "sixth sense," which could lead us to suppose that by consciously employing regular use of essential oils in a loving relationship our sixth sense could be developed, making it easier to "pick up" what our lover needs and wants. In this way it could be possible for couples utilizing aromatherapy and consciously developing their appreciation of natural fragrances to become more "tuned in" to each other, and therefore more able to anticipate each other's sexual needs.

Just as our natural body secretions signal to our mate that we are in the mood for sex, so we could use certain essences in the same way. If, for example, rose or sandalwood oil were used during lovemaking and became associated with making love to one's partner, then after a period of time it should be possible to initiate lovemaking by wearing the scent of sandalwood, and so forth, so that whenever we wanted to precipitate a "night of passion" we could use the same essence to elicit the desired response. Why use an animal pheromone, such as the recently marketed *Boar Mate*, when it is not a pig that we want to attract but a caring and sensitive human being? Why not use sandalwood, which closely mimics the body's natural pheromone and is therefore a sexual attractant, but which was also used in Tantric practice for its spiritually uplifting, as well as its erotic, qualities?

Not Just Behind the Ears

He really bathes
In a large gilded tub, and steeps his feet
and legs in rich Egyptian unguents;
His jaws and breasts he rubs with thick palm oil,
and both his arms with extract of sweet mint;
His eyebrows and his hair with marjoram,
His knees and neck with essence of ground thyme.

Antea Antiphanes

The modern perfume houses, in order to increase their sales revenue, provide a complete range of toiletries in the same fragrance, and although this consistency of smell is "safe" and sophisticated, it is rather boring for lovers, as the nose becomes satiated with one aroma after only twenty minutes. Just as a multiflavored meal can continually titillate the taste buds right down to the last mouthful of food, your body too can be fragranced with different subtle yet erotic aromas, keeping your partner's sense of smell fully alert to the different nuances emanating from various parts of your body.

Anointing different body parts with a variety of fragrances is an art that has been practiced throughout history in many different civilizations. The ancient Arabs believed that four parts of the body should be perfumed: the mouth, the nose, the armpits, and the genitalia. The Romans not only applied aromatics to the hair but to the whole of the body–even to the soles of the feet. The most refined copied the Grecian epicure practice of using a different perfume for each part of the body.

Today we have a far greater choice of essences than any past civilization, and our choice can depend either purely on smell, on the physiological action of an aroma, or on both together.

> Lovers of the past drenched their bodies and their hair in scent; they scattered it over their floors, burned it in their rooms; they wore scented gloves and scented clothes; they bathed in perfumes. They wore rings that ejected spurts of scent on their lovers as they bent to kiss their hands; they pressed their lovers' lips to scented nipples, cupped liquid perfume in their navels and generally indulged themselves in aromatic fantasies.

Leslie Matthews, *The Antiques of Perfume*

Dip into history for the essences that will inspire your lover's pleasure. Remember to keep the fragrancing subtle, as your partner's nose is going to be in very close proximity. Create a feast of aromas–remembering that the nose quickly tires of just one. Be adventurous–perfume the hair, the lips, the nape of the neck, even the feet if you so choose–just remember to choose essences that are safe to use on the skin and only apply those essences to the genitals that you know are harmless to mucous membranes (see chapter 8).

Diluted rose oil is perfect on the nipples–the choice of whether to dilute it with water or camellia oil is up to you.

To scent your pubic hair subtly, apply a little neroli or patchouli to a small soft bristled hairbrush (kept specially for this purpose) and brush through.

Your thighs can be perfumed with dilute vetivert or patchouli; use jasmine around your waist or to anoint your navel, clary sage for your upper chest or neck, and sandalwood oil for your genitals.

Myrtle is slightly rubefacient, which means that it brings heat to wherever it is applied–a little diluted myrtle may be applied to the inside of the thighs or to the labia, and is particularly appropriate to use in this region as, according to Greek lore, it was myrtle which the love goddess Aphrodite used to hide her nakedness. For the dilution, use no more than 2 or 3 drops to a teaspoon of fatty oil.

Black pepper is also a rubefacient oil and may be used in the same way as myrtle, or a tiny amount can be incorporated into a massage oil for use on the genitals. It has a warm, spicy aroma and blends well with several other oils (see chapter 8).

In ancient Egypt perfume was used extensively—well over a hundred different perfume formulas were known, and were used both as camouflage for body odors and as sexual lures.

In Tantric practice, before sexual intercourse the woman is worshiped as the embodiment of the creative force—Shakti. Her body parts are then anointed with different perfumes to honor her creative role and lift up her psyche so that she can manifest as a goddess. In the "Rite of the Five Essentials" (so-called because all five senses would be aroused), the finest oil of jasmine is applied to the hands, oil of patchouli to the neck and cheeks, essence of amber or hina musk to the breasts, extract of spikenard to the hair, musk from the musk deer to the genitals, oil of sandalwood to the thighs, and essence of saffron to the feet. For the man, sandalwood oil or paste would be applied to his forehead, neck, chest, navel, sexual region, upper arms, thighs, hands, and feet.

The ancient texts make little mention of mouthwash or of perfuming the lips, and possibly the daily consumption of aromatic food made perfuming the mouth unnecessary. Today, however, our modern dietary habits make a mouthwash occasionally required. A mouthwash has two purposes–to disinfect/neutralize any germs that cause mouth odor and to excite the sense, enabling the user to "breathe the fragrance of the gods." To combine both purposes into one mouthwash, mix one drop of rose with two drops of bergamot (see chapter 8).

Perfume your lips with dilute rose in camellia–it conditions them while tasting and smelling divine.

Fragrant lozenges were preferred to mouthwashes by the ladies of the eighteenth century, and were available from most apothecaries and perfumers. Those who could not afford lozenges sweetened their breath by chewing a small clove. The flavor and aroma of cloves comes from its essential oil content, and even today chewing a clove is the most inexpensive and reliable breath freshener. Cloves are more than just breath fresheners, though: they contain a powerful antiseptic that can heal mouth abscesses and an analgesic that diminishes toothache.

Clove oil irritates the skin and is not recommended for massage, but if 1 or 2 drops are combined with a teaspoon of camellia or other fatty base oil, the mixture will bring a warm glow when massaged onto the genitals.

The Queen of Sheba had a famous love affair with King Solomon. Sheba, also sometimes known as Punt, was a land of many aromatic plants. The Queen traded many aromatic substances with King Solomon, and before returning to her own land she and King Solomon consummated their relationship. In his brilliant book *Scents and Sensuality*, Max Lake takes journalistic liberties with the biblical account of Solomon's meeting with the Queen of Sheba:

> *My lover put his hand to the doorhole*
> *and my body thrilled and moved.*
> *I rose up to my beloved*
> *my hands dripped with myrrh*
> *fingers of sweet myrrh grasped the handle.*

Scenting Personal Items

Wrap a present to your loved one–in fragrance! Choose a strong cardboard box into which your gift will fit, and a day before sending/giving the gift, place a saucer in the bottom of the box onto which you have placed a tissue sprinkled with a few drops of jasmine, rose, or patchouli oil. Close the lid of the box and leave overnight. Next day, remove the saucer and tissue and you will notice that the cardboard has absorbed the fragrance. When placed in the box your gift will thus be wrapped in fragrance. (This is particularly suitable for giving lingerie or a soft toy or a paper product such as a book–however it is *not* suitable for gifts of cigars or foodstuffs.)

In a similar way, it is possible to perfume writing paper so that if you have to be away from your lover for a period of time your letters will not only convey your deepest feelings in words but the scent emitted from the paper will evoke memories of you. Rose is the traditional scent of lovers–from the time of Venus herself; it is the ideal essence with which to scent a love letter.

Scented ink is very easy to make, as long as you don't use the heavier, viscous oils. Ylang ylang or myrtle are very effective and fairly powerful–add sufficient drops of oil to give the strength of fragrance that is pleasing to your nose. As a general guide use 5 drops of essential oil to one teaspoon (or 5 ml) of ink and mix well. Essences particularly suited for scenting ink are geranium, bergamot, ylang ylang, clary sage, and myrtle. Geranium is best when highly diluted (2–3 drops to every 5-ml spoonful is sufficient). Myrtle oil makes a wonderful scented ink when 10 drops are used to each spoonful of ink. As essential oils will rot rubber if they are left in contact with it for a long time, it is inadvisable to use a pump action fountain pen. An old-fashioned "dip in" pen is ideal and can be rinsed in between fragrances, should you wish each page of your letter to smell different!

Lingerie is easy to perfume, and can be given your personal touch simply by adding some aromatic water to the final rinse (see chapter 8). Use those oils that make you feel sexy—add to a bottle of water, shake well, and add a little to the final rinse when washing delicate items by hand. Do not use the very thick oils as they will not mix very well in water, nor dark oils such as patchouli, as they could stain fabric.

Scented bedclothes are extremely sensual and very personal. One simple way to scent sheets is to place the bottom sheet on the bed as normal and then to spray it lightly (a plant mister is good for this) with a mixture of spring water and the essential oils of your choice—neroli and ylang ylang, for example (see chapter 8). Leave exposed to the air for half an hour if the room is warm, longer if the room is cold. Then make the bed in the usual way. Pillows can be similarly scented for a subtle all-over aroma; for a more powerful fragrance take a piece of cheesecloth or other cotton material the same size or slightly smaller than the pillow, sprinkle it with essential oils, and then place inside the pillowcase so that the aroma seeps through. Again, do not use dark-colored essential oils such as patchouli, as staining may occur.

There are several ways of scenting a bedroom—one method would be to use an electrically heated diffuser into which you

45

drop essence of rose, jasmine, myrtle, or whatever oil you choose. Electric fragrancers are the perfect way to scent a bedroom, as they can be switched on an hour before bedtime to welcome you and your lover to bed. Candlelit fragrancers are very popular today, and fairly inexpensive, but must never be left unattended. A simpler method is to apply a drop or two of essential oil to a radiator or a bowl of hot water. The Empress Josephine had a much more long-lasting method of scenting her bedroom—she had its walls impregnated with musk. It is said that to this day tourists visiting her chambers can still smell the fragrance. English ladies of the eighteenth century imbued their chambers with scented air blown from bellows which had been smeared with strong and sensual aromatics such as musk and ambergris.

Scent your wardrobe and chest of drawers with your favorite aromas, so that your fragrance wafts subtly from your clothing as you walk. The simplest way to scent drawers and wardrobes is to make aromatic sachets to nestle among the clothes. Sprinkle essential oils of rose, myrtle, jasmine, or whatever you prefer onto a cotton wool ball and place it inside a greaseproof bag, then prick a few holes in it with a pin. Place in a drawer or hang in the wardrobe.

Still easy to make but requiring a modicum of sewing skill is a silk pomander. Take a 12-cm circle of silk or other light material. Run a basting stitch around the circumference, and in the center place a cotton wool ball which has been lightly sprinkled with essences. Gather up the thread so that the material encloses the ball, and stitch closed securely. Finish off with a piece of thin ribbon with which to hang it from a coat hanger. Use long-lasting scents such as ylang ylang, rose, patchouli, geranium, myrtle, jasmine, frankincense, or sandalwood. Or use sandalwood as a fixative to give staying power to a lighter oil such as neroli, orange, or bergamot.

Sandalwood is a natural fixative in many perfumes because it is thick, heavy, and has a low evaporation rate. As a general rule, those oils that are viscous–thick and heavy–are good fixatives.

Setting the Scene

He slipped four doves, whose wings were saturate with scents all different in kind–each bird bearing its own appropriate sweets–these doves wheeling in circles round, let fall upon us a shower of sweet perfumery, drenching, bathing both clothes and furniture, and lordlings all.

Xenophanes, *The Settler of Alexis* (quoted in Rimmel, *The Book of Perfumes*)

47

The Emperor Nero had an ostentatious taste for perfumes. In the dining room of his palace he concealed small pipes in the walls; as his guests dined these pipes sprinkled them with a fine mist of erotic scents. Roses were the main flower to be used at Roman banquets and were strewn liberally on floors and even stuffed into cushions so that the reclining Roman would be enveloped in a subtle fragrance and melt into the mood of the evening.

The Roman orgies of food and sex are legendary, and although good food can be conducive to "feeling in the mood," making love after eating a large meal can ruin not only digestion but also lovemaking. The energy needed to make love tends to rob energy from the stomach, and can produce bad indigestion, nausea, or even vomiting. The Romans didn't care because they had a *vomitarium* specifically for this purpose—but "When in Rome, do as the Romans do" need not be applied in this instance!

Preparing Your Own Roman Feast

For a Roman feast fit for an Emperor (or just the two of you), spread the table with mounds of antipasto: cheeses, salami, small pizzas, grilled fish, artichokes, olives—whatever food is desirable to you both—and some (but not too much) wine. If it's all on hand you won't have to leave your lover's company for a second to bring more food.

As the Romans loved rose so much, the scent of rose essence should be the major aroma for this meal. Prepare lots of rose water by adding a drop of rose oil to a bottle of water and shaking it vigorously before pouring it into pretty bowls with which to decorate your table. Float a few rose petals in the water–even if you have to buy a rose from the florist and dissect it, the effect is worth it. Use rose essence on strips of ribbon and tie them prettily around chair legs, curtains, and door handles–or drape them over a warm radiator. You don't, of course, have to wear a toga, but maybe something diaphanous?

A Taste of India

All Indian food contains aromatic spices. To create your own aromatic dinner for two, just decide what food you are planning to serve and work the choice of fragrance around that. Spicy Indian dishes (which can be ordered in advance from many Indian restaurants) are really brought to life by the use of Indian aromatics. If you haven't any saffron–flavored rice you can buy fresh lemongrass from many supermarkets instead, as this gives a delicate spicy–lemony flavor to rice. The Hindu word for rose is "gulab," so gulab jamun would be an appropriately aromatic dessert.

49

Many Indian aromatics are considered to be aphrodisiacal–cardamom, black pepper, clove, cinnamon–and all are combined in "chi" (rhymes with high), a spice tea made with sugar, hot milk, and a special blend of aromatics.

For a special and memorable Indian meal, fragrance the dining room with rose, jasmine, sandalwood, and patchouli. Rose water in a pretty bowl–with some rose petals afloat–makes a wonderful centerpiece. Add a little essence to some lengths of ribbon and drape these over the radiator if it is a chilly winter's night. When summer nights invite you to leave the window open, hang some ribbons sprinkled with jasmine oil (or any of the other "Indian" essences) near an open window so that the breeze can gently waft the aroma into the room.

Chinese Jasmine

Jasmine grows not only in India but also extensively in China, so for a sumptuously fragrant Chinese meal make jasmine the central fragrance.

Jasmine oil should be used subtly, as it contains a chemical called indole (which is similar to an ingredient found in feces) and too much of it tends to be nauseating. When used subtly, however, jasmine is an exquisitely sensual fragrance. Make up lots of jasmine water by adding one drop to a large bottle of water, shaking vigorously, and filling little Chinese bowls with

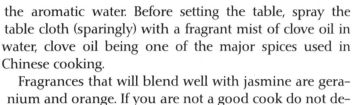

the aromatic water. Before setting the table, spray the table cloth (sparingly) with a fragrant mist of clove oil in water, clove oil being one of the major spices used in Chinese cooking.

Fragrances that will blend well with jasmine are geranium and orange. If you are not a good cook do not despair, as Chinese food can be preordered from a good Chinese restaurant, allowing you to put your efforts into creating a beautiful and loving atmosphere while letting someone else prepare the food. Finish the meal with Chinese jasmine tea.

Sensual Sanctuaries

The Bath

A quiet bath, lit by a gently flickering candle, is a sanctuary from the troubles of the world—a place to relax, to meditate, to let go of troubling thoughts and allow them to drift away as fragrant essences evaporate from the water's surface. Transform the perfunctory habit of cleansing into a ritual of pleasure by adding Aphrodite's beloved myrtle or Venus's rose fragrance and just allowing the aromas to envelop your body and your mind—using the time to think beautiful, sensual thoughts. Even if you can't rationalize why you are loved by your lover–be glad that you are–and if you don't love yourself, because of lack of confidence, fears, negative programming–now is the right moment to start thinking thoughts that will enrich you. Imagine that you are a goddess and fully deserving of love and adoration, and think about what you would like to happen when you and your partner next get together.

By choosing essences of lavender, bergamot, neroli, or geranium you can nourish the very cells of your body while melting away the tensions of the day. To enliven a tired body for a night of passion use essence of rosemary, clary sage, niaouli, or lemon.

A bath is a wonderful retreat for those times when you're not in the mood for sex–maybe you are feeling sad, or worried, or the communication between you and your partner is lacking something–then a long, languorous soak in those healing and energizing essences may just help you to "turn the corner," to feel responsive and be able to adopt a Scarlett O'Hara attitude to those worries–"tomorrow is another day."

The Bedroom

Sometimes a trip into fantasy will be more fruitful than an analytical look at the current problems in your life. Aromatic vapors, massage, gently flickering candles–all can trigger the imagination into a journey somewhere else. Like stepping into an aromatic Tardis, you can leave your troubles behind you and venture into a fragrant world, where aromas of centuries past envelop your olfactory senses and evoke dormant passions. Sandalwood is still the same today as it was thousands of years ago.

> In the pleasure room, decorated with flowers, and fragrant with perfumes, attended by his friends and servants, the citizen should receive the woman, who will come bathed and dressed. At last, when the woman is overcome with love and desire, the citizen should dismiss the people that may be with him. After this, sitting in their own places ... the citizen should apply with his own hand, to the body of the woman, some pure sandalwood.
>
> *Kama Sutra*

Plan an exotic evening of unashamed pleasure. Unless it is the middle of a really hot summer, control your own environment by investing in an electric oil–filled radiator for the bedroom; even if the central heating is off or the rest of the house is just comfortable, the bedroom needs to be about 85°F/30°C,

53

so that being naked for several hours is a pleasurable experience–having to dive under the duvet for warmth is really going to interfere with the fantasy!

Having obtained the desired temperature, the next consideration is the right aroma. Any of the following essences may be used to perfume the room: patchouli, rose, jasmine, clove, sandalwood, cinnamon, cardamom–all are indigenous to India and all are conducive to the fantasy of an Indian summer. Cover the bed with a clean sheet which you have sprayed previously with an aromatic mist, and just allow your imagination to be moved by the heat and the fragrance.

Harem Nights

I know the secrets of love. . . . Throughout the night I give my love call . . . It is I who set the Rose in motion, and move the hearts of lovers. Continuously I teach new mysteries . . . When the Rose returns to the world in summer, I open my heart to joy. My secrets are not known to all but the Rose knows them. I think of nothing but the Rose, I wish nothing but the ruby Rose . . . Can the nightingale live but one night without the beloved?

Fariduddin Attar, *The Parliament of the Birds*

A sign on the bedroom door reads GATES OF FELICITY. Once you and your lover have passed through them into the warm and sensual atmosphere of your "harem" you become each other's slave–"Your wish is my command" or "Speak and it shall be done" may sound like corny lines from *The Arabian Nights*, but spoken by lovers these words open up new experiences and untold joys.

Children love to play "dressing up"–and do any of us really grow too old for this pleasure? Dress up for the evening–harem pants are the obvious choice, and could be outrageously see–through (after all, they are for the eyes of the lover, not for the outside world). An uplift bra, a bare midriff, and silk scarves hanging from a silk pyjama cord tied around the waist would make a passable harem costume. A man's costume might be trickier to manufacture, but a large bath towel tied at the waist would be acceptable.

Bedroom fragrancing should be intensely heavy, as the Sultans liked to show their wealth and power by the copious use of aromatics. Use those essences that both you and your partner are fond of, but use more of them, enough to put you both in the mood for a night of passion.

"Have him stripped and bathed and brought to my tent" is a very powerfully erotic statement! Begin the evening by preparing a sensuous aromatic bath, and be on hand to wash and dry your partner, if so desired. Remember that this is an evening of pleasure and fun, and not to be taken seriously or seen as a precedent for every day. It is like going out to the theatre–enjoy it as a treat.

Bowls of pistachio nuts and grapes or peaches should be placed within reach of the bed for refreshment and sustenance.

The breasts like lilies, 'till other leaves be shared
Her nipples like young blossomed jessamine
Such fragrant flowers to give most odors smell
But her sweet odor did them all excel.

Baudelaire

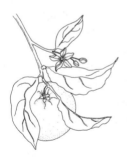

Chapter 4

Massage with Essential Oils

From head to foot with utmost care
Her skin is rubbed with unguents mild,
Fragrant benzoin, oils most rare . . .
And flowers fade in corners there.

Baudelaire

Massage is a wonderful way of being physically close to someone and allowing your loving energy to flow through your hands into your partner. It is also a pleasure to indulge your innate sensuality while benefiting from stress release, relaxation, and general toning. Stress overload causes a breakdown in your immune system, an inability to sleep properly, and a host of other problems. Sigmund Freud recognized that the important things in life are love and work; by massaging your partner one might say you are combining the two.

Still very undervalued and often misunderstood, massage is the key to staying healthy and happy and away from the doctor's office. Much of human behavior is driven by an unending search for renewed pleasurable sensations, and a group of psychology researchers in the United States purport that human beings need most to experience frequent small moments of happiness rather than waiting for the great peaks. Massage is one excellent way of fulfilling this need.

Simple massage plus the correct choice of essential oils can treat problems as diverse as muscular aches and pains, recurrent colds, headaches, and insomnia. A regular massage (once every 2–3 weeks) will enable you to get in contact with your own body, to become more intuitive, and generally to be more resistant to becoming ill.

The spinal column contains nerves that reach every part of your body; massaging the back and applying correct pressure to the spinal area allows these pathways to be kept clear so that energies can flow freely. Massage helps to protect the body by working in harmony with the lymphatic system, which carries off dead cells and poisonous wastes. There are almost 20 liters of lymph in the average adult, and every day about 2 quarts of lymph pass through the thoracic duct, situated along the spinal column. Every time you have a massage, essential oils are passing into the bloodstream and lymphatic system, helping you to become a healthier human being.

You'll not only feel better, but massage makes you look better, too. Frontal massage is perhaps less popular than back massage, but should be enjoyed as well. A very important area to massage is the solar plexus, sometimes called "the pit of the stomach." As well as being linked to our will, the solar plexus is the place of intuition, and is instrumental in the development of psychic power. Diluted rosemary oil rubbed into the solar plexus strengthens the body and gives extra energy when needed, especially when working very long hours, packing up to move, on a long journey with only "junk food" to eat, or when on the receiving end of an outpouring of negative emotion. Rose oil, when rubbed gently into the solar plexus, will soothe the pain of grief and bring comfort in times of sadness and uncertainty.

It may be hard to believe that massage or pressure on the "pit of the stomach" can have a significant effect on sexual potency, or that it can help a man to control his ejaculation; that it can increase the power of "will" and can also release stored tensions from the body. Yet for thousands of years people have recognized this point as being important to their appreciation of sex and life. You do not need to believe it–just try it. You can call it the solar plexus, the third chakra, a shiatsu trigger point, or an acupuncture meridian point. A rose by any other name would smell as sweet.

Preparations

It helps to have had a basic training in massage techniques, but this is not absolutely vital, as long as some basic rules are observed. Your partner should be lying comfortably and you should be positioned to one side of him or her so that you are comfortable and can use your body weight to apply pressure without putting too much strain on your own arms and back. Therapeutic massage can take place on a bed, on pads on the floor, or, of course, on a massage table.

Place a pillow under your partner's ankles and tummy while you are massaging the back, and under the knees while you are massaging the front. Make sure that you have everything on hand that you will need–a massage bowl, massage oil, tissues, and a large towel to cover areas not being worked on. Warm cold hands by immersing them in warm water for a few minutes (rubbing your palms together isn't good enough: your hands may feel warm to you, because you have caused extra blood to come to the surface, but they will still feel cold on a warm back). Also make sure the room temperature is warm and that you and your partner are comfortable and relaxed.

Never pour massage oil directly onto someone, as it will be a shock to the system and not a good start to an otherwise relaxed massage. Pour the oil first into the palm of your hand

and gently rub your hands together so that the oil is evenly dispersed, then apply it to your partner's body.

Therapeutic Back Massage

Place your hands onto your partner at the base of the spine and distribute the oil evenly over the skin. With palms flat and fingers pointing towards the head, glide smoothly up the spine to the neck, then, drawing your hands away from each other, slide them down to the place you started, at the base of the spine. This movement is known as *effleurage* and should be carried out as one continuous movement for at least 10 minutes.

Vary the pressure, and when you find an area that is painful or tender, apply a circular pressure with the pads of your thumbs. Locate and treat all sore areas in this way, remembering to cover exposed body parts with a towel. Complete the massage with another 5–10 minutes of effleurage, making 30 minutes in total. Allow your partner to rest for at least 5 minutes before standing up, and if there is any excess oil on the skin, blot with a towel.

Shoulder Massage

Thousands of people have difficulty getting to sleep at night, and the treatment of insomnia has become a lucrative business for drug companies. Aromatherapy massage is a much gentler alternative. A 10–15–minute shoulder massage given before bedtime, using sedative essential oils, may help your partner to sleep without the need for tranquilizers. If your partner wakes up in the night, a 5–minute massage of the central and upper back area may help them get back to sleep.

Many excellent books exist with detailed instructions in the art of massage, and I'd encourage you to expand your knowledge by further study (see the Recommended Reading section).

Sensual/Erotic Back Massage

Massage is an excellent way to get to know your lover's body. This type of massage differs from a therapeutic one in that it is meant to be a "turn on," not a relaxant as such, although it could be both, of course.

Our skin is designed to process sensation and when we speak of something "touching our heart" it is more than a metaphor; our skin really does speak to our heart. When massaging your lover's back, the main difference from the therapeutic massage is that this massage goes down the back from the nape of the neck to the buttocks and is stimulating rather than relaxing.

Kneel comfortably, facing your lover's feet. After mixing a sensual massage oil, pour sufficient oil into your hand and apply to your partner's body. Begin by placing your hands on your lover's buttocks. The fleshy part of your hand is called "the Mount of Venus" because it resembles the mons pubensis of the goddess. In palmistry this area of the hand denotes levels of sexuality–a weak and flat mount indicating a low sex energy, a fleshy and firm mount indicating a strong and sexual person. The mount is also known as "the heel of the hand," and we should knead the buttocks with this heel of the hand. According to Ouida West in *The Magic of Massage*, "This technique benefits general circulation, the sciatic nerve and the gluteus muscles, which are related to the sexual and reproductive organs."

Next, massage either side of your lover's spine (the same as for therapeutic massage, but this time from the nape of the neck down to the buttocks), using long, languorous caresses. Fondle and knead the buttocks. The buttocks hold a lot of tension, which can be released during this type of massage. Continue these movements for 10 minutes or longer, whatever you and your lover feel comfortable with. This type of massage releases tension that may be an obstacle to lovemaking, and when used in conjunction with stimulation of relevant shiatsu or acupressure points can go a long way towards effecting a cure for impotence or frigidity. (Also see chapter 6.)

Oils to Use

One of the most important oils is the precious sandalwood. Often used for its erotic properties, it can safely be used (suitably diluted) for massaging even the most intimate areas of the body. When massaging the front of your lover pay particular attention to the front of the upper thighs. This area is peppered with acupressure points that tone and stimulate the body, as do the points located in a straight line from the navel to the pubic bone. Incorporate the touching of these important areas into your lovemaking.

All-Over Massage

The ultimate sensual massage has to be the full body massage reputed to be so popular in Bangkok brothels. For this massage both partners have to be naked. Scented oil is applied to your front and/or to your lover's back. With your partner lying facedown, straddle their legs and lean forwards, placing your hands at either side of their body at waist–level (this is one massage where you do *not* use your hands). Slide up and down using your breasts/chest and belly to massage your lover's back. If you feel like it, stop for a moment and, lying on top of your lover, feel the energy between you. Channel your healing energy to your partner if there is a problem for which he or she needs help. Or have fun and write your name on your lover's back using your chin, nose, or nipple. Highly enjoyable in its own right, this type of massage will almost always lead to true lovemaking, but may also be used as a loving gesture if you or your partner feel unable or unwilling to indulge in sexual intercourse.

Shiatsu

Aromatherapy massage is often referred to as being a mixture of Swedish massage and shiatsu. The therapeutic and sensual back massages described above are simple versions of the Swedish method, and here we have a selection of shiatsu "trigger points" that relate specifically to healthy sexual function and may be used on their own or during a complete massage. We can increase sexual vigor indirectly if we stimulate these master points.

Very easy to carry out, shiatsu requires strong thumbs and a desire to help your partner and yourself to enjoy better sexual health. A shiatsu master advises:

> Press with the thumb until the pressure almost turns into pain, then stop and hold this for 7 seconds. Release the pressure until your thumb is just resting on the skin's surface, wait 5 seconds, then repeat 10 times.

These instructions are the basis for treating the following points, with slight variations. The thumb itself should also be massaged, as all of the fingers are intimately connected with the internal organs–particularly the brain. Keeping the fingers strong will strengthen the entire body and, according to the founder of the Nippon Shiatsu School, "energizing the little finger helps to develop a strong heart; shiatsu of the fourth finger helps cure liver trouble; with the middle finger, high blood pressure; index finger for weak stomachs; and strengthening the thumb influences 'the will.' "

Acupressure

Similar to the judo revival points (located just below the collar bones in the middle of the breastbone), the acupressure points can be used to revive a wounded warrior or to tone up the bodies of people whose sexual drives have been assaulted by the judo blows of their modern lives.

Warren and Fischman,
Sexual Acupuncture and Acupressure

Chinese acupressure is very closely connected to acupuncture and makes use of acupuncture points along the meridians. Stimulation of these points encourages the body to heal itself. Acupressure, like shiatsu, can be carried out while the recipient is fully clothed, or it can be incorporated into a massage using scented oils.

There are more than 1,000 specific points along the meridians of the body. It was more than 5,000 years ago that a soldier, shot in the leg with an arrow during battle, discovered that his stomachache had mysteriously disappeared. Over the ensuing centuries this initial discovery was proven again and again and expanded upon until the time of "The Yellow Emperor" (*ca.* 2000 B.C.), who ordered that all medical knowledge be sought out and written down. Much of the knowledge contained in the resultant *Book of Internal Medicine* is still valuable today.

Meridians are channels of energy that flow throughout the body. Each meridian is affiliated with a major organ or bodily function. Several meridians (liver, kidney, and pericordium) have important parts to play, but the two main meridians responsible for the healthy functioning of the sexual organs are known as "the Governor" and "the Conception Vessel": between them these two meridians encircle the body. The Governor begins at the coccyx and travels up the spine and over the crown of the head to end at the center of the top lip. The Conception Vessel starts at the perineum and travels up the front of the body past the genitals, the navel, the center of the chest and up the neck, ending at the center edge of the lower lip. There are many points along these two meridians which, when stimulated, have a beneficial effect on sexual functioning.

Chinese Massage

Chinese massage is similar to both acupressure and shiatsu in that it stimulates the body to heal itself by applying pressure to special points. However, Chinese massage does not confine itself to meridians but works also with soft tissue. Several different techniques are used to obtain good results. Movements such as *pinching* are used to very good effect, as are kneading movements using the knuckles. The Chinese name for the pinching movement is *ning*, and can be an easy movement to master and use for self-massage. Bend the forefinger and middle finger, moving the knuckles together and away from each other.

One of the main points for treating a common cold is the area between the shoulder blades. When treating yourself, it can be difficult to apply the correct shiatsu or acupressure to this area, but it can be "ninged" quite easily.

Another advantage of Chinese massage is that it can be carried out while sitting or standing, whereas for shiatsu or acupressure it is generally necessary for the recipient to be lying down. In addition, Chinese massage can benefit a very fat person, whose acupressure and shiatsu points may not respond.

68

Reflexology

Many external parts of the body have reflexes that affect the internal workings of the body, and this we call *reflexology*. Reflexology is a complex and fascinating therapy in its own right; for our purposes I have only included the reflexology points that affect the sex organs directly.

For a loving couple, the oiling and massaging of the hands and feet is a natural way of communicating, as well as being a basic tool in the art of love.

Two points on the foot are of major importance in the healthy functioning of the sex organs, and are the same for both sexes. The first is the solar plexus area on the sole of the foot, which is located in the center, just below the ball of the foot. The solar plexus, as mentioned earlier, is connected to a person's will. Apply pressure to this area using the thumb. Stimulating this area will energize the sexual organs and help to prevent premature ejaculation in a man.

Premature ejaculation can mean anything from climaxing immediately on entering a woman to not being able to "hang on" long enough to satisfy your partner. Massaging the solar plexus points will help in both cases, but with the latter we must also accept the fact that in general a woman takes longer to arouse and come to a climax than does a man.

The second reflex point is the area on either side of the heel. Massage gently between the thumb and index finger. This area can be very tender but will become less so with regular massage.

Interestingly, these heel points correspond to Achilles' vulnerable spot. According to Homer's *Iliad*, Achilles was the son of Thetis, a sea goddess. When he was first born, his mother dipped Achilles into the holy river Styx, which conferred invulnerability. But the spot on his heel where her fingers held him was not exposed to the magical waters and he was therefore vulnerable in this area. That is why we now describe a weakness or vulnerability in ourselves as our Achilles' heel.

Hand reflexology can be carried out anywhere, anytime–except while driving! You can be massaging your thumbs, and thereby treating your own irregular menstruation or infertility, while riding in a crowded train, at the cinema, and so on–and who's to know?

Massaging the top half, or padded part, of the thumbs will help with menstruation, menopause, or infertility problems in a woman, and impotence in a man. Always give equal attention to both hands. These points are also stimulated when you give a massage to your lover. You could be improving your own sexual functioning by giving your lover a massage!

Massaging the lower outer corner of the Mount of Venus (the fleshy part just below the thumb) stimulates the uterus (or the prostate gland in a man). Opposite the Mount of Venus, on the edge of the palm, is the reflex for the ovaries (or testes).

Ear reflexology, also known as auriculotherapy, is widely practiced in China and other Far Eastern countries. It was instigated a long time ago when it was observed that the shape of the ear corresponded to a baby curled up in the fetal position, and that points on the ear corresponded to parts of the human body.

Facial Massage

Massaging your partner's face is soothing and relaxing for both of you, and puts you in an ideal position for a lingering kiss!

A facial massage also gives you the opportunity to not only massage away the tensions from your partner's face, but also to really get to know this face that you love. The study of the face is known as *physiognomy* and can reveal character traits that you might not have been aware of before. Physiognomy is also a useful means of diagnosis. So while you are caressing your lover's face you can become more aware of his or her state of health, or can use your observations for a character analysis. For example, the shape of the mouth and size of the

lips denote sensuality and generosity, and by study-
ing the jaw line it is possible to see whether your
partner has a strong or weak chin.

Just as a back massage releases tension and in
so doing rids the body of the aging effects of
stress, so too a face massage can remove much
tension and help retain a youthful appearance
while simultaneously benefiting the entire body.

This type of massage can be done at any time as it does not
require the removal of clothing and is an ideal way to help
your partner shed the problems of the day, before those tensions start to spill over. We've all "taken it out" on someone
else when we are feeling angry, frustrated, or negative in some
way. Massaging away those tensions and providing a loved
one with some TLC (tender loving care) will promote harmony
as well as good health.

Facial massage is also conducive to a "Sunday morning lie-
in." No need for formality: just sit comfortably against a wall
or headboard and have your partner lie with her or his head
between your legs. Or sit cross-legged with a small cushion
over your feet, and have your partner place their head on the
cushion. A third option is to kneel behind your partner's head,
facing the feet.

72

Pour a little scented oil into one hand and spread it evenly onto both hands. Place your hands either side of your lover's face and hold gently while you take a few relaxing breaths. Then slowly draw your hands up from the chin to the jawbone, repeating this movement 10–15 times.

Next, draw your fingers across the cheeks from the nose out to the ears–repeat this for a few minutes. Just take your time and enjoy the contact.

Slowly draw the fingers of your right hand across your partner's forehead from left to the right, then draw your left hand across from right to left–this movement needs to be slow and light.

Next, cup your hands under the jaw (with your fingers touching at chin level), then glide your hands up along the jawbone to where the upper and lower jaw meet, applying pressure gently but firmly. Then proceed to massage the points along the jawbone to the chin. There are various "holding points" that should be pressed for a count of five. These can be felt as little indentations.

Continue the facial massage by massaging the area around your partner's mouth, very gently stroking the philtrum (the groove running between the end of the nose and the top of the lip). This area is very sensitive to touch as it is the last of the points on the Governor meridian described earlier and is linked to the part of the brain concerned with sexual function. "It started with a kiss!"

Between the eyebrows and slightly higher up (where a Cyclops' eye would be) is an area that becomes sore if you have not had sufficient sleep, have been thinking too much, or have been overstraining your eyes in some way. Trace a clockwise circle on this part of your partner's forehead and, gradually applying more pressure, make the circle smaller until your finger comes to a standstill in the center. Hold this point for a count of five and release.

Finish the facial massage with more stroking of the forehead and cheeks, and finally use your hands to cup your partner's face—holding for a few moments.

Massaging Your Lover's Head

Without using any scented oil, massage your lover's head as if you were washing the hair. The main points to concentrate on are the crown of the head and the point at the back of the head where the skull joins the neck (the occiput, an important shiatsu point). Just a ten-minute head massage can release a lot of tensions and allow worldly problems to be left outside the bedroom door.

"Since the brain controls sexual activity, this area is of great importance to lovers. A relaxing head massage can quickly alleviate tension, thus opening the body to erotic release" (Ornstein and Sobel, *Healthy Pleasures*).

You could massage your lover's head after a face massage, or a head massage can be carried out at any convenient time of day—now *there's* something to take the mind off of television!

Specific Essences

Essential oils for massage are now widely available to the public via mail order or retail shops. It is important to be absolutely sure that you are using pure essential oils and not a perfumery–grade essential oil, which may contain aromatic chemicals. Although acceptable for the perfume industry, oil of this quality is quite unacceptable for aromatherapy.

Almost without exception the essential oils used in aromatherapy are pleasing to our senses: "we are prompted by a natural instinct to seek and enjoy pleasant odors, and to avoid and reject unpleasant ones" (*Healthy Pleasures*). A few oils, such as tea tree, may be perceived as unpleasant by some people, but because of the unique antifungal and antibacterial qualities of this plant it continues to be used, and rightly so.

Beautiful fragrances inspire us and "while savoring a pleasant fragrance we take slow deep breaths and become relaxed" (*Healthy Pleasures*). We have in an aromatherapy massage oil the perfect accompaniment to a loving massage.

Relaxing oils such as lavender, neroli, and marjoram may be used individually in a suitable diluent or combined together to provide you with an inexpensive but highly effective massage oil. If embarking on the delights of aromatherapy massage for the first time, it is advisable to use one essential oil in a massage base and become familiar with its aroma; observe your partner's response to the fragrance and note how it makes you feel. Gradually build up a small collection of oils and, when you feel confident, make your own massage blends by following the simple tips in chapter 8.

The invigorating oils ravansara, rosemary, and myrtle really do have the power to revitalize a tired or unhealthy body and are particularly good when used after illness.

Rosemary is a very protective and strengthening oil, ideal for massaging into the solar plexus area when we are feeling vulnerable and unable to cope with pressure. Small amounts of lemongrass oil have been proved to be energizing and toning—some professional swimmers have improved on their personal best after a lemongrass massage.

76

"Make love, not war" was the hippie cry of the sixties, echoed perfectly in the lavish use of patchouli oil–a peaceful and erotic fragrance. Patchouli, like sandalwood and vetivert, is an "earthy" aroma and these scents, because of their subtle suggestion of the odor of the reproductive organs, have been used in aphrodisiacal preparations and perfumes for many hundreds of years.

Many aromatic plants mimic closely the aroma of the sexual secretions of the human body–a turn-on in subliminal amounts but a distinct turn-off if encountered in high proportions, so do use these essences sparingly. Sandalwood has been found to contain aromatic molecules similar to those present in semen–the same is true of horse chestnut flowers and or-chids.

Emotional problems and negative emotions can be successfully treated with the use of the uplifting prop-erties to be found in ylang ylang, clary sage, and rose, among other essential oils. Rose oil is wonderfully healing, and when applied to the abdomen will enable you to let go of anger, grief, and sadness. It works on both a physical level (via the skin) and also a more subtle level (via the olfactory sense). If you are suffering from depression (for whatever reason), then ylang ylang or clary sage will uplift and soothe you, enabling you to take stock of the situation in a more objective way and allowing you to take a positive step forward.

Essential oils must be respected if the desired results are to be obtained. For example, if too much of an invigorating oil is used, the effect can be stupor and/or irritated skin–do not be tempted into thinking that if two drops are good then four drops will be twice as good. Many essential oils work best in very low dilutions; too much ylang ylang, for example, will produce a headache, although the use of a few drops can bring fantastic results.

When using essential oils on the genitals, particular care must be taken to use only essences that are not harmful to mucus membranes (see chapter 8). One perfumer related the story of how, as an apprentice, he had disregarded the written notice in the men's bathroom to wash your hands *before* and *after* going to the toilet. Many years later he can vividly recall how the handling of large quantities of lemon oil, and then nonobservance of this rule, caused him two weeks of intense pain, coupled with fear that his "manliness" was going to shrivel and drop off.

When treated with care and a healthy respect, essential oils will provide you with a real therapeutic tool with which to promote healing, enhance sensuality, and enrich your life.

Dos and don'ts for all types of massage:

Dos

※ Do make sure your hands are warm, especially when giving a back massage.

※ Make sure the room is warm before starting a back massage, because the body can cool down considerably during a 30–minute massage.

※ Do remove your watch and any rings that might scratch your partner.

※ Have everything on hand–oil, towels, food, and so on–so that the sensual atmosphere is not interrupted while you go off to find something.

※ Dim the lighting. It is unpleasant to have a bright light shining in your eyes while being massaged.

※ Do take the phone off the hook, switch on the answering machine, or hang a DO NOT DISTURB sign on the door.

※ Enjoy what you are doing. Massage is beautiful.

Don'ts

※ Never use essential oils without first diluting the recommended amount into a fatty oil base.

79

❋ Don't let your partner get cold–use towels to cover up the areas not being worked on.

❋ Never use perfume oils, as they could cause harm. Use only pure essential oils from a reputable supplier.

❋ Don't use essential oils for massage unless you know that they are safe for use on the skin. Some oils, such as clove, will cause reddening of the skin and severe irritation.

❋ Don't worry about getting oil onto bedsheets. A stain remover has been formulated from a blend of essential oils and other natural ingredients. Once rubbed into a greasy spot and rinsed away with cold water, the cloth or sheet can be laundered in the usual way.

Green-myrtled isle where flowers lushly grow,
The quenchless source of all men's veneration,
Where sighs from hearts consumed by adoration
Drift, like the scent of roses as they blow.

Baudelaire

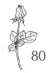

Chapter 5

Beauty Care

Here first she bathes, and round her body pours
Soft oils of fragrance, and ambrosial showers
the perfumed winds, the balmy gale conveys
through heaven, through earth, and all the aerial ways,
spirit divine! whose exhalation greets
the sense of gods with more than mortal sweets.

Homer, *The Odyssey*

A Brief History of Bathing

Aromatic baths and body preparations have been used extensively in many ancient civilizations—the beautifying of the female body made almost an art form.

Scrupulous attention to cleanliness, followed by anointing, shaving, and massaging were of utmost importance to the women of the Arabian harems. These women were renowned for their luminous complexions and satiny skin. Washing and purifying was not only a social necessity but a religious obligation.

The bathing ritual took several hours, often lasting well into the evening. The fashion was for a woman to be smooth-skinned and hairless, so the women would use a depilatory wax made from sugar and lemon juice. After bathing in fragrant waters their skin would be scented with fragrant oils. Rose was frequently used but other popular oils, diluted first in sesame oil, were also in regular use.

To harem women, deprived of so many freedoms, the baths became an all-consuming passion and a most luxurious pastime. The sultan and his wives had private bathrooms, but the other women of the harem shared a large bathhouse. These women of lower rank, who were not wives of the sultan, were known as *odalisques*. *Odalisque* means "woman of the room," which neatly sums up her very limited lifestyle, for when a woman passed through the Gates of Felicity into the harem, there was no turning back.

Today's Turkish baths are an adaptation of the large bathhouses of the harem, which themselves derived from the Roman *thermae*. The shower has of course crept into more and more homes, and the pace of modern living has caused it to take over in popularity. But let's set the record straight: showering is fine for a quick cleanup, but will *never* take the place of bathing as a therapeutic and meditative occupation. A bath scented with essential oils has two purposes–to cleanse the body, ridding it of impurities, and to relax both mind and body.

Japanese bathing rituals have changed little over the centuries, and still remain very much a family affair. The head of the household takes the first and hottest bath of the day and the water is then recycled and reheated until each member of the family has bathed.

Liza Dalby's book *Geisha* explains, "Unless extremely pressed for space, Japanese homes do not have the toilet and bath in the same room. The toilet is given as little space as physically feasible, whereas the luxurious bath is given as much as money and space will allow. Shower attachments off to one side are popular as aids in the process of soaping, scrubbing, and rinsing before getting into the bath itself, but an American–style shower instead of a tub is unthinkable." So important is a relaxing bath after a long arduous day in the office that a Tokyo businessperson can now ring home from the office and electronically program the bath to be run, ready for his or her arrival home.

The "ladies of the night" of ancient Japan kept their pubic hair carefully plucked and clipped, and an experienced man could supposedly "tell the degree of a woman's sexual skill by a mere glance at how she pruned her shrubbery" (*Geisha*).

Shaving your pubic hair is a bold step to take, as it itches a lot and is particularly irritating as it grows back. Trimming your pubic hair into a tidy, groomed shape is very much easier and not at all uncomfortable–it is also very sexy. And because hair retains fragrance, a little "after–trim lotion" can be applied so that a gentle fragrance will emanate from your pubic hair. Whatever your choice of essence–from the delicate floral note of neroli to the heavily sensuous patchouli, you could create your own signature scent.

Today more than ever before we appreciate bathing in scented waters, not only for the sensual delight of inhaling beautiful aromas but because soaking in hot fragrant waters takes away stresses and tensions. With the right essences a bath can be a beauty treatment for the whole body, cleansing and toning the skin, clearing away spots and soothing dry skin, so that thirty minutes after stepping into the bath you can emerge a new person, having left behind the worries and frustrations of the day. Your skin will be delicately scented and silky to the touch and you should be feeling beautiful and loving.

Beautiful Skin, Healthy Body

Our skin is a mirror of our internal health. When the correct oil is chosen both the internal problem and the skin condition will be improved and many skin problems have aromatic solutions.

When the skin is congested the first step on the road to re-covery is an aromatic bath, as essential oils have the ability to decongest tissues and help the body to eliminate toxins. Essence of lavender and essence of rose, being very powerful antiseptic agents but at the same time gentle–acting on the skin, should be used for baths and for massaging affected body parts.

Skin congestion is often symptomatic of poor circulation, as it is the circulating blood that brings a supply of oxygen to the skin cells and keeps them functioning healthily. A rosemary bath or massage will energize body and mind, and because of its stimulant properties will improve the blood circulation and ultimately the condition of your skin.

Chronic skin problems such as eczema and psoriasis may be treated with essential oils of lavender, bergamot, neroli, and rose in a jojoba base.

A spotty complexion is greatly improved by a nightly facial massage with antibacterial essences, and also a regular bathing routine so that your entire body surface is brought into regular contact with dilute essential oils.

Collagen is a protein and is the principal component of connective tissue. When the body suffers from a "connective tissue disease," the underlying symptom is an inflammation–without infection–and is the result of a disorganization of the structure of collagen strands.

Using essential oils to repair and support the health of the entire body may prevent the onset of autoimmune diseases (such as rheumatoid arthritis) that occur when the body no longer recognizes its own proteins and begins to attack its own cells. Prevention is better than cure.

Rose has always been one of the most beneficial essences for a woman's skin, as this story from *The Odyssey* recalls:

> Milto, a fair young maiden, the daughter of a humble artisan, was in the habit of depositing every morning garlands of fresh flowers in the temple of Venus. Her splendid beauty was once nearly destroyed by a boil which grew on her chin, but she saw in a dream the goddess, who told her to apply to it some of the roses from the altar. She did so, and recovered her charms so completely that she eventually sat on the Persian throne as the favorite wife of Cyrus. Since that time the healing powers of the rose have been revered as well as the fragrance.

The rose distils a healing balm,
the beating pulse of pain to calm.

Anacreon

86

Taking Care of Your Face

The beauty of an aromatherapy facial massage is that it works not only on the surface of the skin but also on a deeper level. Essential oils, because of their volatile nature, have the ability to penetrate through the skin to the dermis, the underlying layers of the skin. Essential oils travel through the interstitial fluids, the bloodstream, and the lymphatic system. It is possible to effect a remarkable change in the condition of your skin by applying a treatment oil each night before you go to bed. The massage oil (see chapter 8) should be applied with a gentle massage, using light, upward strokes, and should be left on to work while you are asleep. In this simple way a flawless complexion can be acquired and maintained. Whichever skin type you have, this routine will work for you.

Nature's repair process is slow and steady, with cells being constantly renewed. This cell renewal happens quickly in babies and children and then slows down as we get older. Slower cell renewal means that skin becomes drier, and therefore wrinkles can appear. Dead skin cells are shed more slowly and the skin loses its youthful bloom. By using a nightly aromatherapy facial massage oil we can help the skin cells to renew themselves more frequently, thereby emulating the process of nature when we were young. The removal of dead skin will also create a younger–looking skin, as it is the reflection of light from the skin that denotes a youthful bloom. Conversely, it is the accumulation of dead skin cells on an older skin that prevents this reflection of light, thereby giving the appearance of dull, aged skin.

Dry Skin

Our skin tends to dry out as we get older, and it can look and feel dry and taut. Because of a lack of natural oils, dry skin wrinkles more easily than oily skin and needs daily "feeding" with protective and nourishing oils. Dryness of the visible layer of skin (the epidermis) occurs because the underlying layer of skin (the dermis) is not able to hold sufficient water. You need an emollient to retain moisture in the skin and attract moisture from the atmosphere. Glycerine is commonly used as an emollient for the skin and as a humectant in cosmetics, as it draws moisture from the air. Most people do not require an emollient when air humidity is high, but otherwise one is essential to maintaining a satin–smooth skin.

Jojoba oil is the oil extracted from the desert shrub *Simondsia chinensis*. It is a liquid wax that gives emollience and sheen to skin. Used in conjunction with essential oils such as rose, sandalwood, and vetivert, jojoba can nourish the skin and bring about a youthful look and texture.

Dietrich Gumbel says vetivert "can make the skin feel stout, moisturized and velvety again because fibers of connective tissue swell more easily as well, and are able to bind more water." Sandalwood, another excellent oil for skin care, has been prized since ancient times for the benefit it brings to feminine skins.

A simple skin care routine would begin with cleansing your skin thoroughly. Whereas many commercial cleansers contain detergent or alcohol, which are not good for the skin, you can cleanse your face with a floral water (see below). In the morning a natural moisturizer can be created by leaving a fine layer of floral water on the skin and then applying a tiny amount of night oil. Commercial moisturizers are just a mixture of oils and water combined to form an emulsion.

Dry skin can be caused by other factors besides the natural aging process:

- ❀ central heating
- ❀ overuse of sun beds or sunbathing
- ❀ an imbalance of vitamins and minerals, possibly through an unhealthy diet

- ❀ smoking
- ❀ drinking too much alcohol
- ❀ stress
- ❀ hormonal changes during menopause
- ❀ exposure to strong winds

Floral Waters

A limited number of floral waters are commercially available, but many contain either synthetic aromas or alcohol, neither of which is good for the skin. Make your own very cost-effective and natural floral waters by adding a little essential oil to pure spring water. Essential oils are natural cleansers, and a floral water is ideal for cleansing the face at the end of the day.

Use floral water instead of a cream cleanser to wash your skin; to tone and refresh your face at any time of day; mix with camellia oil to make a "skin vinaigrette" for a fast-acting moisturizer; as a hair rinse after shampooing; and for an eye compress.

You can decide the strength of the floral water, but between 1 and 5 drops for every 100 ml of water is ideal.

Essences that are particularly suited to be made into floral waters are lavender, neroli, bergamot, clary sage, rose, rosewood, camomile, rosemary, and ravansara.

Oily/Acne-Prone Skin

Many essential oils such as lavender, bergamot, neroli, sandal-wood, tea tree, ylang ylang, and lemon are cleansing and anti-bacterial; using one of these will help you to correct a skin infected with acne. Hormone changes during puberty cause the body to produce substances that, if not eliminated quickly by the kidneys and liver, will build up in the body and cause eruptions on the face and neck and occasionally on other parts of the body such as the chest and back. Antibiotics are routinely prescribed for this condition, but can cause more of a toxic build-up. Acne is common among teenagers, especially boys, when the male hormones (testosterone and andro-stenone) become overactive and the estrogen levels are too low, causing too much sebum (a natural oil exuded by the body) to be secreted. This process can be ameliorated with "regulating" essences such as geranium, clary sage, and orange.

When acne is a problem there is always a temptation to apply astringents or to squeeze spots, but both should be avoided as they only stimulate the sebaceous glands and may encourage the spread of bacteria. Instead, cleanse the skin thoroughly with a therapeutic floral water to remove most make-up, surface dirt, and oil, then gently smooth a massage oil for acneic skins into your skin. It will work on a deep level, regulating the secretion of sebum and imparting a natural antiseptic to the infected areas. Used last thing at night, the essential oils will work alongside your own immune system while you are asleep. Very toxic skins will not absorb much oil at first, but when used regularly over a period of time the skin's improvement will be indicated by its ability to absorb more oil. You will not obtain a flawless complexion overnight, but each day you will be working towards an improvement in the appearance and texture of your skin.

Mature Skin

As we grow older our skin cells do not renew themselves as quickly as they once did, which is the reason our skin loses its soft bloom and elasticity. Some essential oils could rightly be called rejuvenators because they have the capacity to speed up the regrowth of skin cells, thereby preserving a youthful–looking, healthy, and soft skin. Rejuvenation is a word that cannot be used in advertising, yet that is precisely what essential oils can do–some essences, such as lavender and tea tree, have the ability to encourage the growth of new skin cells, as illustrated by the many stories of burns and scars being healed by the application of these oils. Other essences that fall into the category of rejuvenators are neroli, rose, myrrh, and frankincense.

Prepare your skin for a nightly massage by cleansing with a floral water and then massaging your face and neck (see chapter 4). To aid penetration of the essences in the massage oil, and to pamper yourself a bit, apply a neroli or geranium compress after your facial massage and then lie down for half an hour or so with your favorite music playing in the background.

A Soothing Compress

Make up a 100-ml bottle of floral water using lavender, neroli, geranium, or camomile, and soak two pieces of cotton wool. Squeeze out the excess liquid and apply the moist pads to your eyes. Lie down for at least twenty minutes.

A compress soothes the eyes of contact lens wearers (but remove your lenses before applying the compress) and is also good for "after-party eyes" when smoke has irritated and inflamed them and possibly given you a headache.

Hips and Thighs

For many women the thighs and hips are the areas of their body they are most unhappy with. Diet alone does not always remove unwanted fat from thighs, but diet along with exercise and using detoxifying and toning essences can make for a big improvement.

Cellulite is the name given to the "orange-peel" appearance of the skin; it is most frequently found on the thighs. It is caused by an accumulation of toxins and fat deposits that should have been eliminated from the body in the normal way but which–because of a sluggish circulation (possibly from sitting at a desk all day)–have settled in the fat of the thighs and buttocks.

Cellulite is a visible sign of congestion not only of the skin but of the organs of elimination. Try a massage of lemongrass oil, which has a draining effect and stimulates the flow of lymph. Lemongrass oil's general ability to fight and eliminate infection in the connective tissues of the body also makes it a valuable aid to slimming, toning, and becoming more resilient.

Cypress oil is an astringent and its use will tone your muscles and improve circulation. Some essential oils such as juniper have a diuretic effect on the body: when used in massage these oils aid the elimination of excess water and toxic deposits. Jojoba oil seems to have the remarkable property of being able to emulsify fats in the deeper layers of the skin, so that the body can get rid of them easily.

Whichever essences you use for slimming and decongesting your thighs, the essences must first be suitably diluted in a fatty base, as a strong concentration will only irritate your skin. Always massage your legs in an upward movement (towards your heart) and keep the strokes firm but not rough. Flesh should never be treated roughly, particularly where cellulite is concerned, because this could make the condition worse.

Legs

For a shiny smooth appearance and feel to your legs, apply a little jojoba after a bath while your skin is still damp. Jojoba also softens dry skin on heels and toes.

Add a drop or two of lavender essence if your skin is irritated or inflamed after shaving or depilation.

Jojoba oil's anti–inflammatory properties make it ideal for treating skin infections, eczema, and psoriasis. It contains Vitamin E in its pure, unbleached form (cold pressed).

Breasts

Small breasts can cause great unhappiness to their owner–and these feelings of insecurity can lead to sexual inhibition. Estrogen is the hormone responsible for developing the breasts–even boys have been known to develop breasts if they use hair lotion containing estrogens.

Some plants–notably geranium, clary sage, and ylang ylang–contain phytohormones (plant hormones). When these oils are used in a camellia base and massaged in every night, it is possible to increase the size of your breasts.

It will take a long time before a significant increase in the size of your breasts becomes apparent, but stick with it. Massage will tone your breasts, and help to stimulate the immune system, so you are keeping yourself in good shape.

Large breasts are the bane of some women's lives, but jojoba oil, because of its emulsifying properties, will help to reduce breast size. When used in conjunction with rose oil (with its astringent properties) regularly over a period of time, it will further minimize breast size.

Hand and Foot Care

The ancient Greek physician Galen is credited with making the first emollient out of beeswax, spermaceti, almond oil, borax, and rose water. Today a simple hand lotion can be made easily and cheaply. Rather like a salad dressing of oil and vinegar, a "vinaigrette" of floral water, camellia oil, and essential oils of lavender, rosewood, and sandalwood will moisturize dry skin on the hands and feet (see chapter 8). This mixture will not keep for long, however, so make it up in small quantities (50–100 ml maximum) and use it within a week or so.

Body Lotion

A simple and effective skin lotion is made by mixing floral water and oil (see chapter 8) and shaking well. Any oil will do–but sweet almond oil was favored by the Romans.

Apply after a bath to keep your skin silky soft and smooth.

Tanning

Having a tan has been the fashion for so many years that per-haps we have forgotten that once it was fashionable for women to stay out of the sun and maintain the same color skin they were born with.

No one should be a "fashion victim," whether this applies to a length of skirt, a particular season's color, or the height of a heel—wear what suits you and what you are happy with. In the same way, whether or not we expose our skin to the sun is a matter of personal choice. Today we encourage people to be proud of their ethnic origins and skin color—except pale-skinned people, who are made to feel that they must be tan to look healthy.

Be true to yourself—if you choose to be "pale and healthy," fine. Choosing to sunbathe is also fine, but take care of your skin because it will age faster when exposed to the sun. Sun-baked skin needs extra nourishment in the form of fatty oils and essences, and you need to drink extra water when sun-bathing.

Jojoba has a sun-protection factor of 4, making it suitable for people who tan easily. Jojoba is also ideal for after-sun care, and with the addition of some lavender oil will protect skin and prolong your tan.

Jojoba oil was used by Native Americans for many skin complaints as well as for treating both dry and oily skin and for protecting and conditioning the hair. Jojoba is a wonderful emollient and is playing its part in the conservation of the whale, being used in cosmetics instead of spermaceti, a wax taken from the brain of the sperm whale. Jojoba has many properties, some of which are unique. It has the ability to emulsify fat and to tone the tissues–ideal for use while dieting or exercising to lose weight. Jojoba is thought to be antiallergenic, which means that it is safe to use on even the most sensitive skins.

Hair Care

O tresses curling round your neck so fair!
O locks! O subtle perfumes I inhale!
Rapture! To fill tonight our secret lair
With memories asleep within this hair;
I long, in the air, to shake it like a veil!

Baudelaire

It is said that bald–headed men are more sexy than other men and this may well be true, but healthy, lustrous hair is the objective of everyone who has a head of hair. Once hair has started to fall out it may be too late to reverse the destructive process. Vital nutrients must be allowed to reach the top of the head; a healthy blood supply must reach the scalp and hair shafts. As stress can be a direct cause of baldness, it is important to reduce stress levels so that your scalp remains a healthy "soil" on which your hair can grow. A head massage is one wonderful way to release tensions and relax the body and mind, while stimulating the scalp and encouraging hair growth.

Aromatherapy hair treatments can recondition hair that has been bleached, permed, or colored. The chosen blend of essential oils mixed into the appropriate fatty base (such as jojoba or almond oil) will feed the roots of your hair while at the same time coating each strand with a fine protective layer of liquid wax. (See chapter 8 for suggestions.)

Dry or Damaged Hair

Adverse weather conditions, perming, coloring, crimping, or even frequent washing with a strong shampoo can all cause damaged hair that lacks luster and feels dry or is splitting. Once every two weeks use an oil treatment to replace natural oils depleted by chemicals or hot sun, to make your hair look better, and to feed your scalp. Massaging your scalp regularly with your fingertips (when you wash your hair and at other times during the day) will aid the circulation of blood and energy to the top of your head and help to promote healthy hair.

For your weekly oil treatment make up a blend of essences (see chapter 8). Pour some of the treatment oil into a saucer or small bowl, and dip in a piece of cotton wool. Part your hair into sections. Apply the oil to the roots of your hair in sections until you have covered your entire head, then, taking more cotton wool soaked in oil, stroke the length of your hair to the ends. Because the very end of the hair is the most dry and brittle make sure that you are generous with the treatment oil. When your hair is saturated, pile it on top of your head and wrap in a towel.

Allow at least two hours before you wash your hair, to ensure that the oil has had a chance to work thoroughly. To get the oil out of your hair, add a little water and work it into an emulsion, then wash your hair in the usual way.

Greasy Hair

Greasy hair is the result of overactive sebaceous glands. It is common during puberty and menstruation. During times of stress, the hair can become excessively greasy, perhaps due to the extra mental pressure of trying to cope. It is almost as if the brain is trying to cool itself down by producing extra quantities of oil. If your oily hair is linked to stress overload, then take steps to relax and calm yourself.

Certain essences have a normalizing effect on sebaceous glands without being astringent and drying the scalp. Tea tree, lemon, geranium, and lavender are some of the oils that would be beneficial in tackling this problem, and at the same time act as safeguards against pimples forming on your scalp.

See chapter 8 for a formula of essential oils for greasy hair. Apply as directed above in the treatment for dry hair, again leaving the treatment on for at least two hours and then washing your hair as usual.

Dandruff

Dandruff usually occurs because of an imbalance of oils on the surface of the skin. Although you might think it is caused by dry skin, it tends to occur as a result of overactive oil glands and often affects people who have acne. Dandruff can also occur as a result of a food allergy, and steps should be taken to try to pinpoint the offending food. Dairy products are the most common foods causing allergy (including Candidiasis–many women suffering from thrush also experience dandruff). If dandruff is accompanied by headaches or a sore neck, a visit to a chiropractor may be useful, as it is easy to suffer a slight subluxation of the spinal bones in the neck.

Even a visit to the hairdresser's, where your neck must support your head while your hair is washed, is sufficient to cause a slight problem.

Although not harmful, dandruff can be embarrassing. Topically, a treatment oil based on jojoba and tea tree oil will greatly improve the condition of your scalp. If there is any fungal growth on the scalp, tea tree is well equipped to deal with it. Its antifungal and antibacterial properties prevent the development of any secondary infections, while dealing quickly and safely with the problem of seborrhea. If you do not like the aroma of tea tree, then jojoba with patchouli or rosemary may be used instead.

Shampoo and Conditioner

It is relatively easy to make your own essential oil shampoo, as there are now several nonperfumed shampoos on the market. Add about 10 drops of essence to every 100 ml of shampoo and mix well. Follow the shampoo with a rinse, using the same essence chosen for the shampoo. A rinse can be made very simply by adding 10 drops of your chosen essence to a liter of water and shaking it vigorously.

For example, you could perfume your hair with the timeless scent of myrtle leaves, in the knowledge that Aphrodite, goddess of love, perfumed herself with the same fragrance. Or use one of the citrus oils of bergamot, lemon, or orange to leave your hair and scalp feeling vibrantly clean and invigorated. Ylang ylang or patchouli rinse poured through your hair after washing will leave a lingering sensual aroma, while rosemary or cypress will strengthen your hair by improving the circulation in your scalp.

In Japan it is not customary to wear perfume, and schoolchildren are forbidden to wear any form of perfume, cologne, or talc, which has caused a trend toward morning hair washing. Every day before school, the girls and boys who wish to smell aromatic wash their hair with their favorite shampoo, which enables them to bypass the school rules without actually breaking them.

To impart an incredible shine to any hair type, take some sweet almond or other nut oil, add jojoba and the essential oils of your choice, and massage through your hair, paying particular attention to your scalp and hair ends, especially if your hair is long and/or split ends are a problem. Arrange your hair on top of your head, cover it with a towel, and leave on for thirty minutes to one hour, then wash off by adding a little shampoo and water to first make an emulsion. Finish by washing in the normal way with a mild shampoo.

A once–weekly conditioning (in the case of dry hair) or once or twice a month (for normal hair) will add a luster that ordinary conditioners don't quite manage, because an

103

aromatherapy conditioner works in an entirely different way from a commercial conditioner. Commercially prepared conditioners are formulated to change the chemical coating of your hair, altering the molecular structure from positive to negative. Although they make your hair look and feel soft and tangle-free, they are of cosmetic use only and do not have much of a beneficial effect on the real condition of your hair. Jojoba, on the other hand, works in a different way. Although the liquid wax does coat the hairs, making them smooth and shiny, there is also considerable benefit to the scalp, and a healthy scalp is the basis for healthy, shining hair. Add whichever essence you most like, but recommended for their sensuous fragrance are rose, patchouli, rosewood, and sandalwood.

Dos and Don'ts

Essential oils are very powerful substances and must be treated with respect. Certain essences should never be used on the skin, and these oils have either been omitted entirely from this book or are accompanied by a warning that they should not be used on the skin (clove, for example). Essential oils are safe to use on the skin providing the following points are observed:

Dos

❀ Make sure that you are using true essential oils, and not a "perfume" labeled as an essential oil. Always buy your essential oils from a reputable company you can trust.

❀ Always dilute essential oils into a suitable base— jojoba, sweet almond, camellia, etc. One to two percent is ample, and many people find that a more subtle blend is more pleasant and equally effective.

❀ For floral waters, shake the essence thoroughly in a bottle of water. Essential oils do not dissolve in water but will disperse sufficiently when shaken vigorously.

❀ Store essential oils away from sunlight. If kept in a bathroom, try to store them in a cupboard where they will not be exposed to steam, as steam, if allowed to penetrate, damages essences.

Don'ts

❀ Never use essential oils directly on the skin (with the exception of dabbing spots with lavender, tea tree, or ravansara, or treating sunburn or a burn lavender). They are highly concentrated, and too strong a dilution could cause irritation to the skin. In order to massage oils into the skin it is necessary to add them to a fatty base so that friction between the two skin surfaces (hand and body/face) is reduced.

❀ Don't use oil such as baby oil (a petroleum by-product) to dilute essential oils, as it will only coat the skin's surface and will not allow the essential oils to penetrate the skin.

❀ Never leave the cap off a bottle of essential oil as the oil will evaporate. Essential oils are highly volatile.

> *When my mind dwells on thee, what a luster assume*
> *All the objects which fancy presents*
> *On my memory thy locks leave a grateful perfume*
> *Far more fragrant than jasmine's sweet scents.*
>
> Moore, *Lalla Rookh Hafiz*

Chapter 6

Achieving Sexual Fulfillment

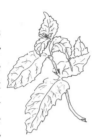

Woman is like a fruit which will only yield its fragrance when rubbed by the hands. Take for example, the basil; unless it be warmed by the fingers it emits no perfume. And do you not know that unless amber be warmed and manipulated it retains its aroma within? The same with woman; if you do not animate her with your frolics and kisses, with nibbling of her thighs and close embraces, you will not obtain what you desire.

Sheik Nefzawi, *The Perfumed Garden*

Making love is beautiful and natural, to be enjoyed and appreciated. Sometimes, though, problems arise that spoil our enjoyment. This chapter looks at how aromatherapy/massage can help. The information given is not intended to take the place of medical advice and attention, but is for people who prefer to use natural treatments whenever possible.

107

For Women

Premenstrual Tension (PMT)

Many women become tense, irritable, and emotional, as well as suffer physical symptoms, a few days prior to their monthly period. Changing hormone levels are responsible for the vulnerability and mood swings common to PMT.

Essences such as clary sage and geranium that regulate the hormones can be used in a bath or in a room fragrancer. Lemongrass is strengthening to the emotions and can either be burned in a room fragrancer or sniffed from a tissue.

Thrush

Genital thrush is a minor health problem but a major inconvenience. It can interfere with enjoyment of sex, make sufferers feel depressed, and, because the accompanying discharge often has an unpleasant smell, can make people very self-conscious.

The usual prescribed treatment for thrush is the use of antibiotic creams and suppositories and although these products do bring temporary relief, the results are very often short-lived and the thrush keeps recurring. Another drawback to using these topical antibiotics is that they kill many healthy bacteria; long-term use can also destroy the balance of bowel flora, which is perfectly balanced in a healthy person (70 percent "good" bacteria/30 percent "bad" bacteria).

Douching

If you have been using antibiotics for thrush and it still has not cleared up, then try douching with warm water and essential oils of lavender, bergamot, ravansara, and tea tree (full recipe in chapter 8).

Purchase a vaginal douche or enema and follow the instructions on how to use it. Add the essential oils to a small, clean bottle; add water. Shake well to disperse the essences, then pour this mixture into the enema bag. Top off with lukewarm–not hot–water.

The number of times you need to douche will depend on the length of time that you have been using vaginal creams and suppositories unsuccessfully. First the douching will wash out any residues of antibiotic cream; further usage will begin a gentle cleansing and healing process.

Two or three daily douches to start with is advisable until there is some relief from irritation; from then on use once or twice a day, especially before bedtime to ensure a comfortable night's sleep. Your partner, even if not showing signs of thrush, should carefully wash the genitals with any of the recommended diluted essences. If you feel a bit depressed, use one of the uplifting essences on a fragrancer in your bedroom or living area, and remind yourself that you are clearing up the problem once and for all.

Essential oils of lemon and niaouli are both highly effective at curing thrush, as each essence has specific properties for genito-urinary problems and also for helping the body to defend itself. Three drops of each essence taken orally on a little brown sugar is the simplest way of using this remedy. Use after breakfast and also before bedtime. However, this is not advisable unless you are sure the essences are pure and unadulterated. If pure, organically grown oils are not available, just use the external treatment.

Thrush, or *Candida albicans*, is a fungal infection, and one of the most powerful antifungal essences is tea tree oil. As well as douching with essential oils, a really bad case of thrush can be ameliorated by inserting into your vagina a tampon soaked in tea tree oil. This simple home remedy will allow you to go about your usual daily tasks without the inconvenience of vaginal itch. Do change the tampon at least three times a day, and douche at night.

Thrush often occurs after taking antibiotics for a more serious genital disease. Finish the prescribed drug treatment and then concentrate on treating the thrush by following the advice given here. Remember to drink lots of mineral water to help your body to eliminate dead cells and antibiotic residue.

Cystitis

This annoying and distressing problem is caused by an infection of the bladder or kidneys. Urinating becomes very painful and the burning sensation is often accompanied by pain further up inside the abdomen.

Sandalwood is particularly suited to treating urinary infections as they are normally caused by bacteria, and in tests sandalwood has been proven to be as powerful as broad spectrum antibiotics in treating many bacterial infections. Rub a little sandalwood onto your lower back (at waist level), where your kidneys are. If your discomfort is very great, have a lavender sitz bath after each visit to the toilet. If this is not practical then add a drop or two of lavender to a small bottle of water and use a swab of cotton wool soaked in the lotion to clean your genital area after urinating.

An alternative treatment for the fast relief of cystitis is to take 1 or 2 drops of juniper berry oil in honey water. It is important that the juniper berry oil is pure, so buy it only from a reputable source.

Vaginal Discharge/Leukorrhea

Vaginal discharge is usually noninfectious and can occur before the onset of the monthly period. This is quite normal, but if the discharge is thicker than normal, has an unpleasant smell, or causes irritation, it could be a sign of something more serious. Sometimes women are allergic to the spermicide used on condoms or with a diaphragm.

Try this simple and effective remedy. Take a tampon out of its protective wrapper, add a few drops of tea tree or lavender oil, and insert. Repeat this procedure at least three times a day. After two or three days, stop using the tampons and see if your discharge has diminished. If you still have a smelly or unusual discharge, then visit your doctor or nearest health clinic.

Vaginal Dryness

Sometimes the vagina secretes adequate lubrication, other times not. Factors affecting this include hormone levels, which fluctuate if you are on the Pill or if your thoughts are dominated by negativity and your emotions are tight.

A simple and effective short-term remedy is to apply a little camellia or jojoba oil directly to your vagina. For the long term, take geranium and clary sage baths, as these two oils are "hormone regulators" and also work on a mental level to harmonize your emotions.

Frigidity

Defined as "lacking friendliness or enthusiasm, dull; (of woman) sexually unresponsive" and "lack or inhibition of sexual feeling, sometimes amounting to aversion," frigidity is difficult to detect. Impotence in a man is easy to spot (no erection), but there is nothing so specific with frigidity.

Because sexual response begins in the mind, there are several essential oils that will lift the emotions and enable a woman to feel sensual. This does not mean, though, that she is automatically going to respond to her partner. For the very reason that sex does start in the mind it can also stop in the mind—if anger and resentment are allowed to brew and are not openly discussed, this will effectively shut down the all-important connection between brain, hormones, and genitals, and instead of an "open" response the reply is likely to be "I'm not in the mood." In his *Taoist Secrets of Love*, Mantak Chia says, "Sex really begins well in advance of the act, as the energies you accumulate then will express themselves when you go deep into sex. Try to calm down any feeling of agitation or anger, as this, more than anything else, will block the flow of energy with your partner and within yourself."

Closing down the emotions to one's partner could easily have the effect of blocking the energy flow to other parts of the body, for example to the hormone system. Testosterone is the hormone primarily responsible for the sex drive in both males and females, and levels of this hormone vary not only between men and women but also among women, with some women producing ten times more testosterone than others. Fear, stress, and anxiety cause the testosterone level to diminish–so use those essential oils that combat anxiety–neroli, rosewood, pine, patchouli, lemon, jasmine, clary sage, or bergamot, in a bath or a massage oil–and use any of the relaxing essential oils, such as rose or lavender, to bring about a relief from stress. Fear may be lessened by massaging rose or rose-mary over the solar plexus area.

Studies have shown that a good sexual appetite seems to help marriage, and that women with high testosterone levels have the best marriages–but how to increase the testosterone levels?

When a man has too much testosterone the outcome is sheer aggression. It would therefore follow that a woman could increase her testosterone levels by sometimes taking on a more "masculine" role–in the bedroom, for instance, by initiating sex and taking a dominant role rather than a passive one. The change itself may be exciting, as getting stuck in any pattern is boring, not only to our conscious mind but deeper, into our psyche.

Boredom is also a factor in the lack of female response–if there is insufficient preparation for her to enjoy the sex act, why should she bother? Why set out for the ice–cream parlor with your partner if he is the only one going to enjoy an ice cream? Eventually you'll think: I can't be bothered–what's in it for me? Jolan Chang, in *The Tao of Love and Sex*, says, "Sex can become mechanical for a man if he forgets or ignores the proper preparation of a woman for lovemaking. Warm the woman with proper foreplay and with warmth of feeling. If you take her body or the sex act for granted the woman will not be properly readied to exchange her love energy through her breasts and lips. If the only contact is genital–penis and vagina, the energy will not flow to the higher heart center, so a man defeats the very goal of what he is seeking if he uses her for a kind of masturbation." Better to stop having sex for a while, and allow the attraction between the two of you to build up again. Explore other avenues–massage, talking, reading erotic prose to each other–all help towards stimulating the many different levels necessary to enjoy the act of love fully. In *Healthy Pleasures* Robert Ornstein says,

> As human beings we are not content, like a dog, to enjoy the same repetitive pursuits, such as going for a walk, having a scratch, chewing a bone. We

constantly are seeking a perfection in our lives, and moving forward towards the goal of happiness. Sexual fulfillment, DIY sex therapy, is one facet of how humans in a regular sexual union can progress to satisfied fulfillment, of pleasing their partners, and receiving the pleasures that they themselves require for happiness. Good sex is the basis of almost all successful marriages, and good sex cannot be boring.

For Men

Impotence

If war's a gamble, love's a lottery
both have ups and downs.
In both apparent heroes can collapse
so think again if you think love is a soft option
it calls for enterprise and courage
take it from me, lovers are all soldiers in Cupid's private army.

Ovid, *Amores*

Temporary inability to achieve an erection can happen to any man at some time in his life. Causes can be physical exhaustion, ill health, the side effects of prescription drugs, or unspoken resentments towards his partner, blocking the flow of energy or chemical messages to the sex organs.

Or perhaps his body is just trying to conserve its store of zinc. Every time a man ejaculates he loses 2.5 mg of zinc, and although zinc is found in many natural foods, if a man is living on junk food then his zinc levels may become very depleted.

Whatever the reason for temporary impotence, it's OK to admit that full intercourse is not going to happen and to be loving and sensual in some other way, such as by massaging your partner. Long-term impotence is most probably going to put strain on a relationship, with your partner thinking you don't love her anymore. Be honest with yourself and your partner and talk openly about what you are feeling.

Research into sex and hormones (as quoted in *Sexual Secrets*) has shown "hormonal secretion is controlled by the pituitary gland, which is situated in the head. Levels of the male sex hormones are increased by exposure to sexual stimuli, but fear, stress and anxiety cause the testosterone level to diminish." Letting go of stress with relaxing aromatherapy massages and baths, and using the shiatsu/acupressure points to strengthen the reproductive system will bring about an improvement. For a man who has been impotent for some time, it may be beneficial to practice penis reflexology each day as well as taking aromatic baths and massages.

Reflexology of the penis is a little-known therapy outside of Taoist love practices and although at present unproven in the West, it would seem to offer a novel and pleasurable way to treat a sexual problem.

Just as there are reflex zones on the hands, feet, and ears, so too on the penis we can find reflexes to the body's internal organs and hormonal system. Using the thumb and fingers, massage (using a circular motion along the shaft of the penis) from the head to the tip and back again. Mantak Chia also asserts that to massage the head of the penis along the prostate reflex is beneficial to the prostate gland and that regular massage can act as a prostate gland cancer preventative exercise.

Readers who wish to know more on this subject are advised to obtain the book *Taoist Secrets of Love* (see Bibliography for details).

Do not forget the power of imagination. Combine your sense of smell with guided imagery. Filling your room with your favorite sensual fragrance–let's say jasmine oil–close your eyes and imagine that you are having a beautiful time with your lover–healing the tensions, giving of yourself. See it taking place in your mind and feel how good it is and how good you feel. Practice these empowering thoughts each day while smelling the fragrance of your choice, until the day it all becomes real and you are cured.

Premature Ejaculation

Next to impotence, the problem men fear most is premature ejaculation.

Tension can be a major cause of premature ejaculation, when there is a sudden buildup of energy in the penis; perhaps the man has not had sex for a period of time or he is tense, especially in the abdomen and buttocks. Have your partner massage these two areas with the relaxing essences of lavender, rose, or geranium; use the strengthening essence of rosemary over your solar plexus. Follow the instructions for treating premature ejaculation by means of "pressure points" (in chapter 4), and if suppressed emotions are to blame then communicate with your partner and allow there to be a flow of energy between you in your everyday lives. Do not wait until you get into the bedroom; make communication part of your daily interaction, part of caring and loving. And love yourself, too—if we are to experience it, we need to believe that we are worthy of love and happiness.

Soreness of the Penis/Scrotum

Soreness caused by irritation of clothing, sensitivity to spermicides, or an accidental scratch can be treated with lavender oil.

119

Sit in a bath to which you have first added 2–3 inches of warm water and 10 drops of lavender oil. Lavender is very healing and will work quickly and safely. If bathing is not convenient, add 4–5 drops of lavender oil to a small bottle of water, shake well, and use cotton wool to apply the mixture to the affected areas.

Problems Both Men and Women Face

Sexually Transmitted Diseases

In many countries in the Western world it is illegal to treat anyone other than yourself for a serious sexual disease such as gonorrhea or syphilis (strangely enough it is not illegal to *give* someone these diseases, only to help him or her get better!). However, over the centuries, people in India and other countries have successfully used sandalwood oil and other plant remedies as a cure for gonorrhea. It may be taken internally– up to 6 drops a day to be taken in a little honey water or on a sugar lump. Sandalwood oil has a bitter taste which some people find unpleasant; therefore "a spoonful of sugar helps the medicine go down." Volume III of *Indian Medicinal Plants* says of sandalwood: "The wood has a bitter taste; tonic to the heart, and the brain; astringent to the bowels, laxative; useful in inflammation, gleet, and gonorrhea."

Sandalwood oil is effective in all genital diseases where there is a discharge of mucus, and its mild analgesic effect helps soothe the pain that often accompanies a venereal disease.

Herpes

Genital herpes is a powerful virus and once it has taken hold it can remain in the body for years to come, tending to flare up when you are under stress or suffering from depression. In other words, it reemerges every time your immune system is low. Building up your immune system is one way to prevent recurrent attacks.

Useful oils for strengthening the immune system are bergamot, sandalwood, tea tree, lavender, niaouli, and ravansara. A weekly massage of your back, thighs, and lower abdomen will help your body to keep the virus under control.

Lack of sunshine can be a contributing factor to an attack, as can depression–so don't sit inside feeling sorry for yourself; use whichever antidepressant oil you particularly like and make sure you get out and about.

Should you be unlucky enough to have a genital lesion, you can treat it with tea tree, niaouli, or ravansara by adding a drop of one oil to the end of a cotton bud, and very carefully applying it to the lesion.

As genital herpes and cold sores of the mouth are caused by the same virus it is very dangerous to indulge in oral sex if either partner has a cold sore. Treat a cold sore the same way you would a genital lesion.

Pruritus

Pruritus means itching and can pertain to the anus or the genitals. It can be caused by external irritation, by wearing jeans or underwear that are too tight, for example, or by the inappropriate use of perfumes or deodorants on these very delicate areas.

Use lavender oil in a sitz bath once or twice a day until the itching has ceased. If dry skin is contributing to the problem, then a little jojoba oil (lightly fragranced with lavender oil) massaged into the area will soothe and heal it (see chapter 8).

Hemorrhoids

Hemorrhoids, or piles, are some of the surest deterrents to sexual intercourse. Hemorrhoids occur when the lining of the rectum swells and is pushed outside of the anus, and can be the result of constipation, overindulgence in alcohol, stress, or even diarrhea.

When even sitting down becomes an agonizing experience it is easy to see that sexual desire could wane considerably.

Aromatherapy treatment for piles is very simple and effective. The two oils to remember are lavender and cypress. Cypress is very astringent, and just a drop or two in a sitz bath

122

(see chapter 8) twice a day has been known to cure piles in a day or two. If cypress is not on hand or you can't tolerate the smell for some reason, then lavender will suffice.

Lavender in water may also be taken to work, or while traveling, and a pad of cotton wool moistened with this lotion may be used after each visit to the lavatory. Even if passing a stool brings tears to your eyes, at least you have a soothing remedy to look forward to and the knowledge that your problem will not last for much longer.

Changing Biorhythms

Sometimes we have more enthusiasm for being physical with our partner than at other times. Our constantly changing biorhythms mean that on some days we may experience an increase or decrease in any one of our three biorhythms: mental, physical, or emotional. Each of the three separate rhythms has a high, low, and critical point every month. Depending on the position of these rhythms we may feel tired, energetic, emotionally strong, emotionally weak, mentally dull, or acute. These rhythms are taken very seriously in Japan, where airline pilots are not allowed to fly on critical days, as the risk of error is greater at this time.

Biorhythms also affect our sexual response, not only toward our partner but toward our own needs and expectations. On a "physical low" day a woman may not feel the necessity to have

123

an orgasm, just being content to be in close contact with her lover, whereas on a "physical high" day she could be a raging lust–machine. Emotions are also affected by bio–rhythms, so when you're having an "emotional low" or "critical" day, use aromatherapy oils to strengthen and uplift yourself.

Fear or Embarrassment About Oral Sex

Because we are taught in school that "sex" is when a man and a woman have intercourse, his penis entering her vagina, and as this is presented as the goal of sex, it becomes a focus for most adults. But the art of lovemaking, as well as perhaps involving the union of the sex organs, also incorporates union of the lips, union of intertwined bodies, and union of the mouth with the genitals.

Fear of how another person may perceive her genital aroma causes many women to shun cunnilingus. Yet it is a pity to deny oneself the pleasures and joys of this intimate form of loving expression just because of negative associations.

As a prelude to lovemaking, have a vaginal douche with a fragrant and sensuous essence (see chapter 8) to thoroughly cleanse your vagina, in the same way that you clean your teeth and use a mouthwash to be sure of the wholesomeness of your breath. To convince yourself that your own body perfume is attractive to your partner, why not take some vaginal fluid and dab it on your left shoulder, or in the middle of your chest, and see if your lover has a preference for that area. Courtesans of medieval Europe attracted customers by using their sexual secretions as perfume, behind their ears and around their necks. It is interesting to note that Camembert and Brie cheeses have a smell reminiscent of the vaginal odor, which itself is sometimes referred to as "cheesy." If your partner does not like cheese or has a "sweet tooth," you could apply a little homemade rose water or a little neroli in honey to your "yoni" (see chapter 8).

Some women have an aversion to or fear of fellatio, or "playing the flute" as it is referred to in Eastern books of love. The genital aroma of a freshly bathed man should not be a turn-off, as nature intended this aroma to be a sexual turn-on. Perhaps earthy smells do not get you excited and you prefer the sweeter, more ethereal fragrance of flowers? In that case why not add a little floral fragrance to your lover's bouquet? Take care to use only those essences that are nonirritating, such as rose, neroli, and ylang ylang and make sure that they are very diluted.

Sandalwood, above all others, is the perfect aromatic for genital use. It may be diluted in jojoba or camellia for a delicate fragrance, or it may be used alone. More information on this wondrous oil can be found in chapter 3.

In India and China oral sex has always been considered a normal part of the art of loving, and in an Eastern book called *The Golden Lotus* we find a sweet poem about "the playing of the flute":

> *Not from bamboo or stone, not played on strings,*
> *This is the song of an instrument that lives ...*
> *Who can say what the tune is, or the key?*

Side Effects of Prescription Drugs

While most sexual difficulties are usually no more than a transitory hiccup, if they persist the worry can lead to the physical disorder becoming a psychological one. Stress and illness are two common causes of sexual dysfunction, yet how many people would ever suspect prescription medicines of being responsible for their problem? Medicines can upset libido or other aspects of sexuality through their effects on the glandular and reproductive system, muscle tone, or even simply by causing drowsiness or depression. The male reproductive system is also sensitive to chemical influences and some drug side effects can amount to chemical castration. While taking medicines men may experience changes in libido, difficulty in obtaining or sustaining an erection, an inability to ejaculate normally, decreased levels of testosterone resulting in swelling or shrinking of the testicles or penis, a lowered sperm count, or the development of breasts.

According to Gill Martlew ("Can Medicine Ruin Your Sex Life?" *Living*, October 1989) some drugs to be aware of are:

- Antihistamines: Taken to combat the problems of hay fever–as well as the known side effects of drowsiness, these drugs can cause loss of libido in both sexes, and men may experience temporary impotence.

- High blood–pressure drugs: These may decrease desire in both sexes; men may experience impaired erection and ejaculation. Women may suffer impaired arousal.

- Tranquilizers: Diazepam may decrease libido in men and women, and men may experience difficulty in achieving an erection.

- Tetracycline: This drug, which is commonly prescribed for acne, can produce inflammation of the vagina, causing discomfort during intercourse.

- Birth control pills: Can cause a decrease in libido and decreased vaginal lubrication, causing discomfort during intercourse.

Complementary Remedies

The following remedies are available from most health food stores and can enhance the body's natural state of health, necessary to fully enjoy making love.

Zinc

Zinc is vitally important to healthy sexual functioning and although other factors must be taken into consideration, zinc deficiency can be the cause of impotence, depression, mood changes, and subfertility.

The authors of *The Zinc Solution* say "even a very slightly lowered zinc status could mean a sperm count too low for reproduction to take place. It can also lead to loss of libido and even impotence." Zinc has been found to be necessary for the development of healthy sperm and "in subfertile men the numbers of spermatozoa have been found to be related to the zinc content of the seminal fluid."

Zinc is found naturally in many foods and as long as a man is eating a healthy diet, there is probably no need to be concerned about zinc levels in the body—however, as 2.5 mg of zinc is lost in every ejaculation, if a man is not eating properly then not only is he impairing his fertility but he is putting his long-term state of health at risk. Zinc is important to the functioning of the immune system, and a prolonged deficiency of zinc can lead to a malfunction of the thymus gland, which is the body's major production site for lymphocytes.

Women also need zinc, especially during their childbearing years, but as women do not lose zinc from the body in the same way as men do, zinc supplementation is not so vital.

Echinacea

Echinacea is an herb indigenous to North America. It would once have come under the heading of a "blood purifier," but today would be classed an "immunostimulant." Fifty years of research into the properties of Echinacea have proved that it is a nonspecific stimulant to the immune system, which verifies the Native American claim that it has more healing properties than any other plant. Taken each day echinacea helps to enhance the body's resistance to infection and works in tandem with essential oils to protect your long-term health.

Increasingly taken by people to reduce their allergic reactions to certain foods—such as dairy products—echinacea may be of use to hay fever sufferers who experience a loss of libido due to taking antihistamines.

Guarana

If you are recovering from an illness or jet lag, or if you just need to sustain long-term physical exertion, Guarana (with its active ingredient, guaranine) will tone your body.

Caffeine is made from the Guarana seed, but only after roasting it, which changes its chemical structure and significantly alters the natural way in which Guarana works. Guarana works synergistically, unlike caffeine, as it contains many other ingredients that combine to bring gentle tonic properties to the body, releasing muscle tensions while sharpening the mind.

Particularly useful for all cases of weakness and debility, both physical and mental, using Guarana regularly promotes a sense of well-being. Users may find that less sleep is needed—useful when embarking on a "night of passion." Tests carried out by acupuncturists show that after taking Guarana for a short period, a person's meridian energies become balanced and blocked energy is released. This would perhaps account for the claims made about its aphrodisiacal properties, as any blockage in the meridians of the sexual organs may inhibit the body's natural sexual response.

Catuaba

Catuaba, harvested from Brazil, is a useful adjunct to any aromatherapy treatment for impotence, as it is a tonic for the genitals. It stimulates the nervous system and is known on its native soil as a natural aphrodisiac and sexual stimulant. Cat-uaba tea needs to be taken regularly for a period of time before its benefits are experienced–including the onset of erotic dreams, followed by an increase in sexual desire.

Heightening Your Pleasure

Kissing

Kissing is an important facet of lovemaking for several different reasons and has been written about at length in the *Kama Sutra*.

Most obviously, the lips and tongue "echo" the labia and the penis. Stimulation of the meridians connecting the lower lip to the genitals and the upper lip to the "sex center" of the brain is probably the reason why we were born with two fleshy protuberances above our chins with which to "kiss" our partner. Prolonged stimulation of the lips will release the necessary sex hormones and awaken the energies that normally lie inactive and, like a dormant volcano, suddenly burst into activity.

According to the ancient Chinese sex manual *The Art of the Bedchamber*, a man is like fire and a woman like water. The fire easily flares up but the water takes a longer time to heat. Kissing is a necessary and very pleasurable part of any foreplay.

Saliva has many properties that are invigorating for lovers, and if we think about a dog and how it will lick its wounds until healed, we can see that saliva has healing properties. According to Taoist books, the exchange of saliva harmonizes the Yin and Yang within each partner.

The art of kissing can be made even more pleasant and sensual by the use of aromatic mouthwashes and the application of a scented lip balm (see chapters 3 and 8).

Contraception and Aromatherapy

Condoms

Condom use is increasing with the necessity of safe sex but still does not have a general following among fertile couples. Other forms of contraception used by women, such as the diaphragm and the Pill, continue to win the popularity stakes.

In Japan the situation is different, and condoms are used by almost 80 percent of fertile couples. To a nation of people concerned with harmony, the idea of taking chemicals that interfere with the hormonal system and cause an imbalance in Yin and Yang is considered unacceptable. Condom distribution is more widespread in Japan and they are sold in packs of 25, 50, or 100, making them an economic method of birth control.

As well as the expense, one of the major drawbacks to the popularity of condoms is that they are considered to be too dry and to have an off-putting, rubbery smell. And some people find that the spermicide used in condoms causes irritation. Although most condoms contain spermicide, there are some manufactured without, and these are generally known as *hypoallergenic*. If in doubt, ask your pharmacist for advice.

While researching and writing this book I conducted my own tests into the compatibility of dilute essential oils with condoms. Some were filled with water and then rubbed with dilute essential oils; others were blown up like balloons and subjected to the same test methods. Finding the condoms intact after several days, I assumed that there was no damage to the condoms. However, having spoken to LRC Products Ltd., makers of condoms, their advice to me was that oil-based products should never be used with condoms, as a weakening of the latex could result. As my own experiments were nonscientific, I must bow to the superior knowledge of LRC and their exhaustive testing methods and recommend that readers do *not* use essential oils or fatty oils with condoms.

Honey Cap

The diaphragm is a popular female contraceptive because, like the condom, it is a "natural" product, being made from rubber, and need only be used "as and when." It does not interfere with the body's chemistry, but it *can* interfere with the spontaneity of sexual response as it needs to be inserted prior to sexual intercourse and removed again within eight hours.

Its other drawback is that it has to be used in combination with a spermicide, which can cause allergic reactions in sensitive people.

A new and smaller diaphragm has entered the market in the last few years that has all of the advantages of the regular diaphragm but none of the drawbacks. Known as the *honey cap*, this diaphragm really is a natural product, as the rubber is impregnated with honey, a natural spermicide. When not in use you keep it in a pot of honey and as honey is antibacterial, this is the only form of protection it needs. The honey cap need only be rinsed in lukewarm water before insertion, and may be left in place for up to seven days at a time. While being worn it is perfectly all right to bathe and swim, allowing a woman much greater freedom, and taking an aromatic bath or having an aromatherapy massage is quite safe. However, never let undiluted essential oils come into contact with the honey cap as this could cause the rubber to perish and the contraceptive would no longer be reliable. When used correctly, the honey cap has been found to be as effective as a condom in preventing pregnancy.

Many a flower reluctantly
Spills its fragrance secretly
In deep and hidden solitudes.

Baudelaire

Chapter 7

Aroma and Sexual Response

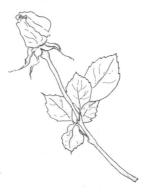

They haven't got no noses
the fallen sons of Eve
even the smell of roses
is not what they supposes
but more than mind discloses
and more than men believe.

G. K. Chesterton

As we have seen, aroma plays a fundamental and profound role in human sexual response.

The most rudimentary knowledge of animals, insects, birds, and even flowers and plants demonstrates that nature uses "sexual attraction" to ensure the continuation of a species. Peacocks flaunt their beautiful tails, flowers attract the bee by color and scent, many animals have a mating call or a ritual dance. What we may not be aware of is the powerful effect of smell (although most of us will have noted the "nose–to–tail" greeting behavior among dogs, for example) and that some female animals in heat produce an odor guaranteed to excite the requisite response in the male.

As human beings we do not generally like to be reminded that we are animals. We feel that we possess qualities, attributes, and powers that raise us above animal responses–yet however true this may be, we produce "sex–attractant chemicals" just as animals, insects, and plants do.

Interestingly, the most celebrated perfumes contain these sex attractants: musk and civet from animals, jasmine and sandalwood from plants. How and why they work has remained somewhat mysterious, but in the latter half of this century many perfume companies and universities around the world have embarked upon extensive research into the mechanisms of aroma and our sense of smell.

One researcher into the psychology of perfumery, Joachim Mensing, says,

> A few decades ago the functional meaning of the limbic system [an area of the brain] was totally unknown and was simply described as "the smelling brain." Today, however, we know that this limbic system serves as the central circuit for emotions, moods, motivation, and sexual behavior. It can be

136

stimulated directly through the sense of smell. Furthermore, the limbic system also plays a significant role in selecting and transmitting information between our short- and long-term memories. Selection from, and transmission to, these two memories is performed via corresponding associative regions of the limbic system. The limbic system receives its information from the various sensory regions, such as the sense of smell.

The links between smell, hormones, and sexuality are quite fascinating, if somewhat complex. Rather than try to reach a conclusion, the reader is invited to browse through the following "aroma information":

33 Olfactory Facts

1. Every person has an individual scent signature.
2. Our emotions, health, and diet all affect our body odor and the smells we find pleasant. This explains why the same perfume smells different on different individuals, and why we can grow to dislike perfumes we once loved.
3. Our mood–be it happy, angry, or frightened–and personality–extrovert or introvert–contribute to our total scent.

137

4. It may be difficult to accept the relationship of emotion, personality, and odor. But odor can make you happy, hungry, angry, drowsy, depressed, frigid or impotent, or sick. Each mood has an odor–happiness, for example, is an odor improver. You can smell happy.

5. Happy hormones–beta endorphins–are produced by babies who are massaged, cuddled, and stroked, and these babies have higher survival rates. These happy hormones are made by the body whenever you achieve a terrific result after hard mental or physical effort or are deeply moved by natural beauty, art, or music.

6. PEA (phenylethylamine) is found in both rose water and chocolate. It is the chemical thought to be responsible for the "rush" felt when falling in love.

7. Without knowing it, people communicate sexual attraction to one another in greater or lesser degree by scent. This fact has been recognized since time immemorial, but waited until thirty years ago for a name. *Pheromone*–from the Greek for "transfer" and "excitement"–describes the substance, usually volatile, produced by one person that evokes a response in another.

8. Most of us remain unaware of how our sense of smell influences our passions. We may be attracted to or put off by people we meet yet be unaware that this is in part because of the way they smell.

9. When a Frenchman or -woman is repulsed by someone, he or she uses the expression, "Je ne peux pas le sentir," which means literally "I can't stand his smell."

10. Pheromones are an invitation to mate and are secreted by the sex glands, in vaginal secretions and saliva, and via the skin.

11. One of the drawbacks of birth control pills is that they rob a woman's bodies of copulins, the special sex scent of her sexual secretions which play a large part in stimulating the male sex drive.

12. Androstenone, the principle male pheromone, is produced by special glands (apocrine) that empty on the hairs. It is formed in both sexes by the influence of testosterone. It smells of musk and is the raw fuel of libido. It drives the female menstrual cycle.

13. One third of the population can't smell androstenone. It can provoke aggression in men. Men

139

who have been castrated do not produce any androstenone.

14. During puberty, scent glands in eyes, ears, mouth, nose, head, armpits, sex organs, and anus are developed and their secretions become especially active. The scent glands' secretion increases also in adults during sexual excitement. These substances are also called pheromones.

15. Female pheromones can be diffused across a room, but male pheromones can only be transferred by intimate contact.

16. Male pheromones, which are discharged from special sweat glands in a man's armpits and around his nipples and genitals, can only be transferred by intimate contact, i.e., during sex.

17. There is evidence that the pituitary acts as an inner extension of the nose, relaying the nose's messages to the gonads via a system of hormones.

18. The odors of sandalwood, the pig-mating pheromone (*Boar Mate*), and human axillary secretions are remarkably similar.

19. All the sexual fragrances can be alluring at olfactory threshold levels, or possibly even below.

This means that these scents are perceptible even when very dilute.

20. Humanity's loss of the need to "smell danger" has led to the development of the sense of smell for sensual purpose.

21. About one person in six cannot detect the odor of semen–pyrroline.

22. Humans have more scent glands than any other higher primate, and women have higher numbers than men.

23. Research has shown that high estrogen levels–occurring just after ovulation and during pregnancy–correlate with increased olfactory awareness, which can actually cause nausea and morning sickness.

24. Smell is the most subtle sense. All smells register at very low levels of intensity . . . intense flavors and perfumes may have an instant appeal at one time or another, but they produce rapid fatigue, sometimes in seconds, to be followed by indifference, then aversion and, if intense enough, vomiting.

25. The area of the brain associated with smell directly stimulates the limbic area of the brain,

which controls our emotions, memory, sex drive, and intuition. The olfactory area of the brain also connects with the hypothalamus, which controls the hormonal system by influencing the "master gland," the pituitary.

26. The nose contains ten million neurons that catch odor molecules. These are called *olfactory receptors*. They send odors to the emotional center of the brain.

27. We can experience pleasure through our eyes, ears, nose, and mouth, but we can also experience it through purely mental means; we can stimulate the pathways of the limbic system with a flow of positive, optimistic messages from our higher cortical brain centers.

28. More is being learned about smell and memory. Suppressed memories can be revived by particular smells associated with childhood, etc., and good "vibes" (happy hormones) can be encouraged with attractive aromas.

29. The olfactory membrane is the only place in the human body where the central nervous system is exposed and in direct contact with the envi-

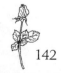

ronment. The cells of the olfactory membrane are brain cells.

30. The olfactory mucosa, which lines the narrow olfactory slits, has a structure analogous to the spongy central body of the penis and is equally erectile.

31. Erectile tissue is found in only three parts of the human body: the genitals, the chest, and the nose.

32. Many people suffer from "honeymoon rhinitis" whereby the nose runs all the time. This is because the nose lining swells during sexual stimulation.

33. No one really knows how the olfactory cells in our noses work, but recently three American scientists put forward the theory that the cells operate not chemically but by recognizing the size and shape of the molecules of a substance. In the receptor cell there are submicroscopically small apertures of various shapes and sizes, into which fit the equivalently shaped molecules. It is rather like the toddler's game of fitting plastic shapes into a toy letter box. Spherical molecules

register as the smell of camphor, discs as musk, tailed discs as undifferentiated flowers, wedges as peppermint, and rods as ether. All smells are made up from these basic ingredients, rather as all colors can be made from the primary colors.

> *The horizon all around me*
> *breathed out perfume*
> *announcing her arrival*
> *as the fragrance precedes a flower.*

Colin Franzen (ed.), *Poems of Arab Andalusia*

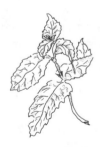

144

Chapter 8

Essential Recipes

*Scents are surer than sights and sounds
to make your heart strings crack.*

Rudyard Kipling

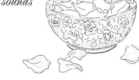

The recipes given here are cross–referenced to the chapters in which they are described. There is also a table at the end of this chapter providing an at–a–glance list of the essential oils discussed in greater length in the book.

For all of these recipes I have mentioned camellia oil as my preferred fatty oil (used to dilute the other essential oils). Acceptable alternatives to camellia oil include sweet almond, safflower, peanut, and grape seed oils. I find camellia oil preferable because it does not oxidize–therefore your mixtures will keep without going rancid. If you will only be using the oils occasionally, this is worth bearing in mind. Also, because camellia oil has virtually no scent of its own, it will not interfere with the aromas of your chosen essential oils.

For similar reasons I have suggested that, where water is used to dilute the oils, you use spring water rather than tap water. Essences last longer in spring water.

Where jojoba oil is mentioned specifically as the base oil, it is because only jojoba will achieve the required results.

Vetivert oil is very beneficial to the skin and has an earthy aroma, making it the perfect oil to use for sensual massage. It is expensive, however, and because of its powerful scent only minute amounts should be used. I would recommend no more than 1–2 drops to 100 ml of camellia oil. This vetivert dilution may be used as the basis for a massage oil for the face or body, with the addition of the essences mentioned in the appropriate recipes, below.

Note: I am confident about taking essential oils internally because I buy organically grown oils, mostly from the grower or agent of the growers, in the country of origin. However, I am concerned about the purity of many of the essential oils on sale in the stores. *Please* use for internal use only essential oils that have been organically grown, are pure and unadulterated, and have been tested for purity prior to sale to the store. Many of the essential oils sold are not pure enough for internal use and should not be used for this purpose. In France, where many doctors prescribe essential oils for internal use, there are very strict controls over the purity and freshness of essential oils sold through pharmacies. Sadly, there are no such controls in the United States and "essential oil" companies can sell any quality oil to the public. Please beware.

Chapter 1: Aromatherapy for Life

Goddess Bath

6 drops myrtle to a full bath
Swirl water with your hand to distribute the oil through the bath water. People with sensitive skin may wish to use fewer drops and/or add the oil to a small bottle of water, shake well, and then add to the bath.

Nourishing Bath

2 drops lavender
2 drops bergamot
2 drops neroli
1 drop geranium

Enliven-a-Tired-Body Bath

1 drop niaouli
2 drops rosemary
2 drops clary sage
1 drop lemon

147

Harmony Bath

5 drops geranium
5 drops clary sage

Add to a deep, hot bath to harmonize the emotions and regulate hormones.

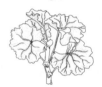

Chapter 3: Lasting Impressions

Oils Safe to Use on Private Parts

Rose or sandalwood (diluted in camellia oil or vetivert).

Rubefacient Oils

A rubefacient oil can be used to bring a gentle heat to an area of the body (a safe and aromatic equivalent of the aphrodisiac Spanish fly).

Myrtle: 2–3 drops diluted in 1 tsp of camellia oil
(or other fatty oil)

Black pepper: 1–2 drops in 1 tsp camellia oil

Black pepper also blends well with sandalwood and rose: add 1 drop of each of these three oils to 2 tsp camellia oil.

Clove oil: 1 drop to 1 tsp camellia oil

Note: Clove oil is very powerful and should not be used by anyone with skin allergies.

Scented Mouthwash

1 drop rose
2 drops bergamot

or

1 drop clary sage
2 drops orange

Add oils to a 100-ml bottle of spring water. Shake well.

Scented Lip Balm

1 drop rose
1 tsp camellia oil

Store in small, tinted glass bottle.

Scented Ink

Take the oil of your choice. Add 5 drops of it to 1 tsp ink.
Geranium-scented ink: 2–3 drops to 1 tsp ink.
Myrtle-scented ink: 10 drops to 1 tsp ink

Scented Lingerie

Add 10 drops of your favorite oil to a 1-liter bottle of spring water. Shake well. Add enough of this mixture to the final rinse of a machine (or hand) wash to impart the amount of fragrance you desire. *Note:* Do not tumble dry the lingerie after the wash, as this will cause the fragrance to evaporate.

Scented Bedclothes

Take ylang ylang, neroli, or the oil of your choice. Add 2 drops to a 500–ml bottle of spring water. Shake well. Pour into a plant sprayer and spray a fine mist over the bed–clothes. For a more pronounced fragrance, just add a few more drops of oil to the water.

Scented Bowls for a Table Setting

Add 2 drops of either rose, jasmine, orange, or geranium to a 500–ml bottle of spring water. If you'd like to use clove oil instead, add just 1 drop to 500 ml water. Shake well. Pour into pretty bowls and place these on the dining table.

Chapter 4: Massage with Essential Oils

For the following recipes, the number of drops of essence recommended can be adjusted according to your particular preferences. If you are very fond of one aroma, use a drop more than is recommended. If you are not as enamored of a scent, use a drop or two less. Let your nose be your guide.

Soothing Sleep
3 drops marjoram
2 drops geranium

2 drops lavender
1 drop neroli
30 ml sweet almond or camellia/sweet almond mix

Sensual Massage

2 drops sandalwood
2 drops clary sage
1 drop ylang ylang
Either 1 drop jasmine or 1 drop rose (as an optional extra)
30 ml "vetivert base" (see page 146) or sweet almond oil

Energizing Massage for Body or Mind

2 drops rosemary
3 drops bergamot
1 drop ravansara
2 drops myrtle
30 ml sweet almond or camellia/sweet almond

For the Solar Plexus

3 drops rose or rosemary
2 tsp camellia oil

You can make up a lot of this dilution and keep it handy for those times you want to feel replenished: Add 1 ml rose or rosemary to 100 ml camellia oil. This amount will last a long time.

For the Immune System

10 drops of sandalwood, tea tree, lavender,
niaouli, ravansara—alone or in combination
2 tsp sweet almond oil
Massage into the back and upper chest (armpit to armpit
and up to the base of the neck).

For the Genitals

1 drop rose
1 drop sandalwood
1–2 tsp camellia oil
Vetivert dilution (1–2 drops only to 100 ml of camellia
oil) can be used in place of pure camellia oil.

Hand and Foot Massage

2–3 drops oil to 2 tsp camellia oil:
Peppermint for hot feet
Myrtle for cold feet
Cypress for smelly feet
When recovering from an illness, a soothing foot or hand
massage can be made with any of these oils: niaouli,
lavender, ravansara, bergamot, lemon, neroli, rose.

Chapter 5: Beauty Care

Sluggish or Blemished Skin

To decongest the skin, bathe in lavender and ravansara, adding 3 drops of each to the bath. Make up a massage oil to use on the back, upper chest, face–wherever your skin has become congested and/or spotty:

3 drops bergamot
3 drops ravansara
3 tsp camellia oil

Blemish (Spot) Treatment

Put a drop of lemon, eucalyptus, tea tree, lavender, niaouli, or ravansara on a cotton bud and apply directly to the spot.

Facial Massage Oils

Antibacterial Blend for Acne-Prone Skin

2 drops ravansara
2 drops lavender
2 drops ylang ylang
Either 2 drops lemon or 2 drops bergamot

20 ml camellia oil
10 ml jojoba

Rejuvenating Blend for "Thirty-Something" Skin

1 drop neroli
2 drops lavender
2 drops geranium
3 drops sandalwood
15 ml vetivert base (see page 146) or plain camellia
10 ml jojoba
5 ml rosehip seed oil (optional)

(If the rosehip oil is not used, just add 5 ml more of camellia oil.)

Beautifying Blend for Normal/Dry Skin

2 drops ylang ylang
2 drops rosewood
2 drops lavender
2 drops sandalwood
10 ml jojoba
15 ml camellia oil
5 ml rosehip seed oil

Rosehip seed oil is excellent for treating dry or mature skin and can rightly be called a rejuvenator. However, it is not suitable for oily or blemished skin.

Cleansing Lotion/Floral Waters

You can use floral waters to cleanse and tone the skin on your face and neck. Use any of the following essences (1 drop to 100 ml spring water): lavender, neroli, ravansara, rosewood, camomile, bergamot, clary sage, geranium, niaouli. This mixture can also be used to clean the genitals. If you prefer a more subtle aroma, add 1 drop essence to 200 ml spring water.

Facial Compress

To soothe tired, sore eyes:
2–3 drops lavender or neroli to 100 ml spring water
or 1 drop camomile to 100 ml spring water

Skin Vinaigrette

For silky smooth, sensuously fragranced skin:
5 drops myrtle, ylang ylang, patchouli, clary sage, neroli, jasmine, or rosewood
20 ml camellia oil
100 ml spring water

Shake well. Alternatively, use 100 ml floral water (see above), 20 ml camellia oil, and a drop or two of chosen essence; shake well. *Note:* This mixture will resemble salad dressing in that the ingredients will separate if left to stand–always shake well before use.

Anti-Cellulite Formula

Once a week, massage the problem area with the follow-ing blend of essences:

> 1 drop lemongrass
> 1 drop cypress
> 1 drop juniper
> 1 tsp jojoba

On other days of the week, use lavender in jojoba (1 drop in 1 tsp) to massage into the cellulite.

Breast Care

To tone and enlarge:

> 2 drops geranium
> 2 drops clary sage
> 2 drops ylang ylang
> 2 tsp camellia oil or vetivert base

This will make enough massage oil for a week or so. If you find the aroma too strong, just add more camellia oil.

To tone and reduce:

> 1 drop rose
> 1 tsp jojoba

Massage this blend into the breasts. Jojoba emulsifies fat tissue, while rose is astringent.

After-Sun Care

To soothe the discomfort of too much sun:
> 5–10 drops lavender or tea tree
> 100 ml spring water

Shake well. Splash on; soak a handkerchief and use as a compress; pour into a plant sprayer and spray on.

> 5–10 drops lavender
> 2–3 tsp jojoba

This mixture will nourish the skin while protecting and prolonging your tan.

Hair Care

Jojoba and almond oil or jojoba and camellia oil may be used as the base for each of the following once–a–week treatments to condition your hair:

Normal Hair

> 1 drop rosewood
> 1 drop lemon
> 1 drop rosemary
> 3 tsp base oil

157

Dry and Damaged Hair

1 drop geranium
1 drop lavender
1 drop orange
3 tsp base oil

Greasy Hair

1 drop lemon
1 drop cypress
1 drop juniper
3 tsp base oil
or
1 drop patchouli
1 drop ylang ylang
1 drop lavender
3 tsp base oil

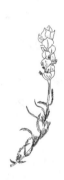

Dandruff

5 drops tea tree
3 tsp base oil (a pure jojoba base is very good at
fighting dandruff)

158

Essential Oil Shampoo
10 drops myrtle
or
5 drops rosemary
5 drops lemon
or
Up to 10 drops of the essential oil(s) of your choice
100 ml nonperfumed shampoo

Hair Rinse
For sensual–smelling, shiny hair:
5 drops bergamot
2 drops lemon
3 drops orange
or
2 drops ylang ylang
8 drops patchouli
or
Up to 10 drops of the essence(s) of your choice
1 liter spring water

To make a strengthening rinse for thinning hair:
6 drops rosemary

159

4 drops cypress
1 liter spring water
Unused rinse may be kept indefinitely.

Chapter 6:
Achieving Sexual Fulfillment

Therapeutic Douche

Up to 10 drops of one or a mixture of these essences:
Lavender
Bergamot
Ravansara
Tea tree
100 ml spring water
Shake well; then add to enema pot and top off with comfortably warm water. Use once or twice a day for thrush, heavy vaginal discharge, or irritation until the condition clears up.

For Genito-urinary Problems

3 drops lemon
3 drops niaouli
a little brown sugar

Apply the oils to the sugar and eat. *Note*: Never take oils internally unless you are quite sure of their purity.

Cystitis Remedy

1–2 drops juniper berry
honey water: ½ tsp runny honey
a little hot water

Mix ingredients in a glass. Drink. Cystitis will normally improve after 24 hours or so, but if the problem has not cleared up within a week, discontinue treatment and seek medical advice.

Lavender Sitz Bath

Add 10 drops lavender to a large bowl (large enough to sit in) or to 2 inches of warm water in the bath. Mix thoroughly. Sit for 10 minutes or so. Alternatively, swab the genital area/anus with cotton wool dipped in lavender water.

Hemorrhoids (piles) can be treated by adding 10 drops cypress to a sitz bath. Mix well by stirring your hand through the water before you sit in it or add the cypress to a small bottle of water, shake well, then add to the sitz bath.

Aromatic Tampon

To treat thrush, irritation, vaginal discharge: 5–10 drops tea tree or lavender. Apply to the tip and sides of a tampon. Change the tampon at least three times a day.

Healing a Sore Scrotum

4 drops lavender
4 drops tea tree
100 ml spring water

Bathe the affected area.

Treating a Genital Lesion

Tea tree
Niaouli
Eucalyptus
Ravansara
Lavender

Add a drop or two of one of these oils to a cotton bud and apply directly to the lesion. This treatment may also be used for a cold sore.

Gonorrhea Remedy

6 drops sandalwood
brown sugar or honey water (see above)

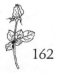

162

Mix ingredients and swallow or drink. Continue taking this mixture once a day until the condition is improved (but for no longer than three weeks).

This treatment is not meant to replace a visit to a clinic for sexually transmitted diseases (STDs), but to be used afterwards, perhaps before having to resort to antibiotics.

If the problem has not cleared up within three weeks, then take the antibiotics.

There is no adverse reaction between sandalwood oil and orthodox medication, so it is worth pursuing the gentle treatment first.

Celibacy is always advisable when you are trying to clear up a sexual disease.

Sensuous Douche

To cleanse and fragrance the vagina:

5–10 drops of one or a mixture of these essences:

Rose

Neroli

Ylang ylang

Bergamot

Geranium

100 ml spring water

163

Shake well; then top off douche or enema pot with comfortably warm water.

Anointing the "Yoni" and "Lingam"

1 drop rose
100 ml spring water

Shake well before use.

or

1 drop neroli
2 tsp runny honey
1–2 tsp water

Blend well so the mixture is thick but liquid.

or

1 drop rose
1 tsp runny honey
1 tsp water

or

1 drop rose
1 tsp camellia oil

or

1 drop ylang ylang
1 drop sandalwood
2 tsp camellia oil

Mix well.

Note: A drop is quite a lot of flavor and for a more subtle taste, just dip the end of needle (darning or tapestry thickness) into the essence and stir into the honey.

> *Tonight we're getting love messages,*
> *For their sake we must not go to sleep.*
> *The fragrance of your hair spreading through the streets*
> *Make the perfumers wonder at such competition.*

Rumi, *Unseen Rain*

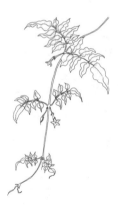

165

	bergamot	black pepper	camomile	clary sage	clove	cypress	eucalyptus	geranium	jasmine
air fragrancing	●				●			●	●
bath blends	●		●	●				●	●
mouthwashes	●				●				
lip balm									
scented ink	●	●		●				●	●
scented lingerie	●							●	●
scented bedclothes	●			●				●	●
therapeutic massage	●	●	●	●				●	
sensual massage		●		●					●
energizing massage	●			●				●	
solar plexus massage									
hand and foot care									
facial oils	●		●	●				●	
facial compress			●						
floral waters	●		●						
cellulite						●		●	
breast care				●					
after-sun care									
hair care			●					●	
hair rinse			●					●	●
douches	●								
genito-urinary problems									
internal remedies				●					
sitz bath						●			
hemorrhoids						●			
aromatic tampon									
yoni/lingam fragrancing		●							●

jojoba	juniper	lavender	lemon	lemon grass	marjoram	myrtle	niaouli	orange	orange blossom (neroli)	patchouli	peppermint	ravansara	rose	rosemary	rosewood	sandalwood	tea tree	ylang ylang
			●			●		●	●				●		●			●
	●	●	●		●	●	●	●	●				●	●	●	●		●
			●				●	●	●		●		●				●	
										●			●					
						●			●				●		●			
						●			●				●		●			●
						●		●	●				●		●			●
	●	●	●	●	●	●	●	●	●				●	●	●	●	●	
●						●	●		●				●			●		●
			●	●		●	●	●						●				
													●	●				
		●									●		●			●		
●		●	●						●				●		●	●	●	●
		●							●				●		●			
		●							●				●		●	●		
●	●	●		●									●			●		
●													●					●
●		●														●	●	
●			●			●			●					●			●	
						●		●					●	●				●
		●					●						●				●	
	●		●				●									●	●	
	●		●				●				●					●		
		●															●	
		●																
		●															●	
						●	●		●				●			●		●
						●			●				●	●		●		●

167

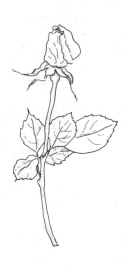

Glossary of Essential Oils
Their Common and Latin Names

Bergamot   *Citrus bergamia*
Black pepper   *Piper nigrum*
Camellia   *Camellia*
Camomile, roman   *Anthemis nobilis*
Clary sage   *Salvia sclarea*
Clove   *Eugenia caryophyllum*
Cypress   *Cupressus sempervirens*
Eucalyptus   *Eucalyptus globulus*
Frankincense   *Boswellia carterii*
Geranium   *Pelargonium graveolens/roseum*
Jasmine   *Jasminium grandiflorum*
Jojoba   *Simmondsia chinensis/californica*
Juniper   *Juniperus communis*
Lavender   *Lavandula angustifolia*
Lemon   *Citrus limonum*
Lemongrass   *Andropogon citratus*

Marjoram (Spanish)   *Thymus mastichina*
Myrtle   *Myrtus communis*
Niaouli   *Melaleuca viridiflora*
Orange   *Citrus auranthium (fruit)*
Orange blossom (neroli)   *Citrus auranthium (flowers)*
Patchouli   *Pogostemon patchouli*
Peppermint   *Mentha piperata*
Ravansara   *Ravansara aromatica*
Rose   *Rosa centifolia*
Rosemary   *Rosmarinus officinalis*
Rosewood   *Aniba parviflora*
Sandalwood   *Santalum album*
Tea tree   *Melaleuca alternifolia*
Vetivert   *Andropogon muricatus*
Ylang ylang   *Canangium odoratum*

Bibliography

Altman, Nathaniel, *Sexual Palmistry* (The Aquarian Press, 1986); reissued as *Palmistry for Lovers* (1993).

Bornoff, Nicholas, *Pink Samurai* (Grafton, 1991).

Bryce–Smith, Derek, and Liz Hodgkinson, *The Zinc Solution* (Century Arrow, 1986).

Burton, Richard (trans.), John Muirhead–Gould (ed.), *The Kama Sutra of Vatsyayana* (Grafton, 1963).

——. Sir Richard Burton (trans.), Charles Fowkes (ed.), *The Illustrated Kama Sutra/Ananga Ranga/Perfumed Garden* (Hamlyn, 1987).

Chang, Jolan, *The Tao of Love and Sex* (Wildwood House, 1977).

Chia, Mantak (with Michael Winn), *Taoist Secrets of Love* (Aurora Press, 1984).

Croutier, Alev Lytle, *Harem (The World Behind the Veil)* (Bloomsbury, 1989).

Dalby, Liza, *Geisha* (Vintage, 1983).

Douglas, Nik, and Penny Slinger, *Sexual Secrets, the Alchemy of Ecstasy* (Destiny, 1979).

"Fragrance Special," *Marie Claire*, 1991.

Fromm, Erich, *The Art of Loving* (Mandala, 1985; originally published 1957).

Gallway, Timothy W., *The Inner Game of Tennis* (Cape, 1975).

Gumbel, Dietrich, *Principles of Holistic Skin Therapy* (Karl F. Haug, 1986).

Hindu Myths (Penguin Classics, Penguin, 1975).

Junemann, Monika, *Enchanting Scents* (Schneelowe, 1988).

Kirtikar, K. R., *Indian Medicinal Plants* (Int'l Book Distributors, 1986).

Lake, Max, *Scents and Sensuality* (John Murray, 1989).

Manaka, Y., and I. A. Urquhart, *Chinese Massage* (22d printing, Shufonotomo Ltd, 1988).

Martlew, Gill, "Can Medicine Ruin Your Sex Life?" *Living*, October 1989.

Matthews, Leslie, *The Antiques of Perfume* (G. Bell & Sons, 1973).

Namikoshi, Tokujiro, *Shiatsu* (Japan Publications, 1972, 1983).

Nefzawi, Sheik, *The Perfumed Garden*, Sir Richard Burton (trans.), Alan Hull Walton (ed.), (Grafton, 1963).

Ornstein, Robert, and David Sobel, *Healthy Pleasures* (Addison–Wesley, 1989).

Pullar, Philippa, *Consuming Passions* (Hamish Hamilton, 1970).

Rawson, Philip, *The Art of Tantra* (Thames & Hudson, 1978).

Rimmel, Eugene, *The Book of Perfumes* (Chapman & Hall, 1865).

Stoddart, D. Michael, *The Scented Ape* (Cambridge University Press, 1990).

Thompson, C. J. S., *The Mystery and Lure of Perfume* (Bodley Head, 1927).

Walker, Barbara G., *The Woman's Encyclopedia of Myths & Secrets* (HarperSanFrancisco, 1983).

Warren, Frank Z., and Walter Ian Fischman, *Sexual Acupuncture and Acupressure* (Unwin, 1978, 1980).

West, Ouida, *The Magic of Massage* (Hastings, 1986).

Woolger, Jennifer B., and Roger J. Woolger, *The Goddess Within: A Guide to Eternal Myths That Shape Women's Lives* (Fawcett, 1989).

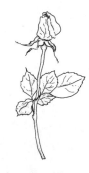

Recommended Reading

Davies, Rodney, *How to Read Faces* (The Aquarian Press, 1989).

Dawes, Nigel, and Fiona Harrold, *Massage Cures* (Thorsons, 1990).

Foster, Steven, *Echinacea: Nature's Immune Enhancer* (Healing Arts, 1991).

Inkeles, Gordon, *The Art of Sensual Massage* (Thorsons, 1992).

Kunzi, Kevin and Barbara, *Hand and Foot Reflexology* (Thorsons, 1984).

Lavabre, Marcel, *Aromatherapy Workbook* (Healing Arts, 1990).

Lundberg, Paul, *The Book of Shiatsu* (Gaia, 1992).

Tisserand, Maggie, *Aromatherapy for Women* (Thorsons, 1985, 1990).

West, Ouida, *The Magic of Massage* (Century Hutchinson, 1983).

West, Peter, *Biorhythms* (Thorsons, 1980).

Woolger, Jennifer Barker, and Roger J. Woolger, *The Goddess Within* (Rider, 1990).

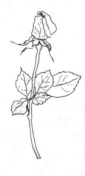

Index

177